Acupuncture for Pain Management

Yuan-Chi Lin • Eric Shen-Zen Hsu
Editors

Acupuncture for Pain Management

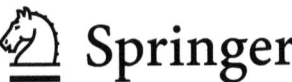

Editors
Yuan-Chi Lin
Director, Medical Acupuncture Service
Senior Associate in Perioperative
Anesthesia and Pain Medicine
Department of Anesthesiology,
Perioperative and Pain Medicine
Boston Children's Hospital
Associate Professor of Anaesthesia
(Pediatrics)
Department of Anaesthesia
Harvard Medical School
Boston
Massachusetts
USA

Eric Shen-Zen Hsu, MD
Pain Management Fellowship
Department of Anesthesiology
David Geffen School of Medicine at UCLA
Los Angeles, CA, USA

UCLA Pain Management Center
Santa Monica-UCLA Medical Center and
Orthopedic Hospital
Santa Monica, CA, USA

ISBN 978-1-4614-5274-4   ISBN 978-1-4614-5275-1 (eBook)
DOI 10.1007/978-1-4614-5275-1
Springer Heidelberg Dordrecht London New York

Library of Congress Control Number: 2013946429

© Springer Science+Business Media New York 2014
This work is subject to copyright. All rights are reserved by the Publisher, whether the whole or part of the material is concerned, specifically the rights of translation, reprinting, reuse of illustrations, recitation, broadcasting, reproduction on microfilms or in any other physical way, and transmission or information storage and retrieval, electronic adaptation, computer software, or by similar or dissimilar methodology now known or hereafter developed. Exempted from this legal reservation are brief excerpts in connection with reviews or scholarly analysis or material supplied specifically for the purpose of being entered and executed on a computer system, for exclusive use by the purchaser of the work. Duplication of this publication or parts thereof is permitted only under the provisions of the Copyright Law of the Publisher's location, in its current version, and permission for use must always be obtained from Springer. Permissions for use may be obtained through RightsLink at the Copyright Clearance Center. Violations are liable to prosecution under the respective Copyright Law.
The use of general descriptive names, registered names, trademarks, service marks, etc. in this publication does not imply, even in the absence of a specific statement, that such names are exempt from the relevant protective laws and regulations and therefore free for general use.
While the advice and information in this book are believed to be true and accurate at the date of publication, neither the authors nor the editors nor the publisher can accept any legal responsibility for any errors or omissions that may be made. The publisher makes no warranty, express or implied, with respect to the material contained herein.

Printed on acid-free paper

Springer is part of Springer Science+Business Media (www.springer.com)

To my wife, Eva, for her love, support, and sacrifice.
To my daughters, Katerina and Josephina, who bring joy to my life.
To my mother, Mrs. Chu-Niang Lin-Sung, and in loving memory of my father, Dr. Chen-Chuan Lin, who guided me toward the path to passion, wisdom, and responsibility.

Yuan-Chi Lin

Preface

The book *Acupuncture for Pain Management* features practical information for incorporating acupuncture into the practice of pain medicine. It is written for clinicians interested in integrating acupuncture into pain management.

Part I sets the foundation for practicing acupuncture. It includes the history of acupuncture, basic theories and pattern discrimination in Traditional Chinese Medicine, mechanisms of acupuncture analgesia, common acupuncture practices, peri-operative acupuncture, acupuncture pain research, and auricular acupuncture. Part II addresses acupuncture Qi flow, point measurement, the twelve acupuncture principal meridians and extrameridian points. Part III presents the practical aspects of acupunture pain management for common pain and realted conditions, including headache, facial pain, vertigo, toothache, neck pain, chest pain, epigastic pain, abdominal pain, dysmemorrhea, upperback pain, scapular pain, low back pain, sacroiliac joint pain, coccygeal pain, shoulder pain, elbow pain, wrist pain, hip pain, knee pain, ankle pain, heel pain, insomnia, nausea, vomiting, sedation, and dizziness. The editors and authors have worked to ensure that these chapters reflect the need for acupucnture pain management. It is our hope that this book will provide clinicians with a sound foundation in acupuncture and the practical aspects of acupuncture pain management.

The authors, Drs. Yuan-Chi Lin, Yue-Pang Mok, Lynn Rusy, Shu-Ming Wang, Eric Hsu, Tat Leang Lee, and Yung-Fong Sung, are the founding instructors for the American Society of Anesthesiologists (ASA) acupuncture workshop, which was organized and established at the 2002 ASA annual meeting. This book is also an international collaborative effort, with contributions from Drs. Francisco Lozano, Tat Leang Lee, Z Zheng, Jen-Hwey Chiu, Jaung-Geng Lin, Kuen-Bao Chen, and Yu-Chen Lee.

I would like to acknowledge all those who have devoted precious time to make this book a reality. My sincere appreciation goes to my colleagues at the Department of Anesthesiology, Perioperative and Pain Medicine at Boston Children's Hospital. Thanks to my chairman, Dr. Paul Hickey, and to Dr. Charles Berde, Chief of Pain Medicine, whose vision and support helped me establish the Medical Acupuncture Service at Boston Children's Hospital in September 2000.

I give special thanks to Margaret Lyons for her thoughtfulness and editorial expertise, to the staff at Springler, Michael Sova, Jyoti Kalra, Joanna Perey and Shelley Reinhardt for their careful guidance throughout the publication process.

I am blessed to have the most loving and compassionate family. I shall always treasure the values, education, and inspiration I received from my late father, Dr. Chen-Chuan Lin, and my mother, Mrs. Chu-Niang Lin-Sung. I thank the constant encouragement, wisdom and strength I received from my four brothers. Finally, I am most grateful to my wonderful wife, Eva, and my children, Katerina and Josephina, for their unwavering support and unconditional love.

Boston, MA, USA   Yuan-Chi Lin

Contents

Part I General Consideration

1. **History of Acupuncture** 3
   Jen-Hwey Chiu

2. **Basic Theories of Traditional Chinese Medicine** 13
   Francisco Lozano

3. **Pattern Discrimination in Traditional Chinese Medicine (TCM)** 45
   Francisco Lozano

4. **Mechanisms of Acupuncture Analgesia** 73
   Annie D. Lee and Eric Shen-Zen Hsu

5. **Common Acupuncture Practices** 87
   Shu-Ming Wang

6. **Perioperative Acupuncture** 101
   Yue-Pang Mok

7. **Acupuncture Pain Research: Quantitative and Qualitative** 117
   Tat Leang Lee and Zhen Zheng

8. **Auricular Acupuncture** 139
   Yung-Fong Sung

Part II Acupuncture Channels

9. **Acupuncture Qi Flow and Points Measurement** 153
   Yuan-Chi Lin and Cynthia S. Tung

10 **Hand Tai Yin Lung Meridian** 手太陰肺經穴 159
Yuan-Chi Lin and Rosalie F. Tassone

11 **Hand Yang Ming Large Intestine Meridian** 手陽明大腸經穴 161
Yuan-Chi Lin and Rosalie F. Tassone

12 **Foot Yang Ming Stomach Meridian** 足陽明胃經穴 165
Yuan-Chi Lin and Rosalie F. Tassone

13 **Foot Tai Yin Spleen Meridian** 足太陰脾經穴 169
Yuan-Chi Lin and Rosalie F. Tassone

14 **The Hand Shao Yin Heart Meridian** 手少陰心經穴 173
Rosalie F. Tassone and Yuan-Chi Lin

15 **The Hand Tai Yang Small Intestine Meridian** 手太陽小腸經穴 175
Rosalie F. Tassone and Yuan-Chi Lin

16 **Foot Tai Yang Bladder Meridian** 足太陽膀胱經穴 179
Rosalie F. Tassone and Yuan-Chi Lin

17 **Foot Shao Yin Kidney Meridian** 足少陰腎經穴 185
Rosalie F. Tassone and Yuan-Chi Lin

18 **Hand Jue Yin Pericardium Meridian** 手厥陰心包經穴 189
Lynn M. Rusy and Yuan-Chi Lin

19 **Hand Sho Yang Triple Energizer Meridian** 手少陽三焦經穴 191
Lynn M. Rusy and Yuan-Chi Lin

20 **Foot Shao Yang Gall Bladder Meridian** 足少陽膽經穴 195
Lynn M. Rusy and Yuan-Chi Lin

21 **Foot Jun Yin Liver Meridian** 足厥陰肝經穴 199
Lynn M. Rusy and Yuan-Chi Lin

22 **Conception Vessel** 任脈經穴 203
Yuan-Chi Lin and Lynn M. Rusy

23 **Governor Vessel** 督脈經穴 207
Yuan-Chi Lin and Lynn M. Rusy

24 **The Extra Acupuncture Points** 奇穴 211
Yuan-Chi Lin and Cynthia S. Tung

Contents

Part III Clinical Conditions

25 Headache 221
Jaung-Geng Lin, Kuen-Bao Chen and Yu-Chen Lee

26 Facial Nerve Palsy 225
Jaung-Geng Lin, Kuen-Bao Chen and Yu-Chen Lee

27 Vertigo 227
Jaung-Geng Lin, Kuen-Bao Chen and Yu-Chen Lee

28 Toothache 229
Jaung-Geng Lin, Kuen-Bao Chen and Yu-Chen Lee

29 Neck Pain 231
Jaung-Geng Lin, Kuen-Bao Chen and Yu-Chen Lee

30 Chest Pain 233
Jaung-Geng Lin, Kuen-Bao Chen and Yu-Chen Lee

31 Epigastric Pain 235
Jaung-Geng Lin, Kuen-Bao Chen and Yu-Chen Lee

32 Abdominal Pain 237
Jaung-Geng Lin, Kuen-Bao Chen and Yu-Chen Lee

33 Dysmenorrhea 239
Jaung-Geng Lin, Kuen-Bao Chen and Yu-Chen Lee

34 Upper Back Pain 241
Jaung-Geng Lin, Kuen-Bao Chen and Yu-Chen Lee

35 Frozen Shoulder 243
Jaung-Geng Lin, Kuen-Bao Chen and Yu-Chen Lee

36 Low Back Pain 245
Jaung-Geng Lin, Kuen-Bao Chen and Yu-Chen Lee

37 Arthritis, Joint Pain 247
Jaung-Geng Lin, Kuen-Bao Chen and Yu-Chen Lee

38 Coccygeal Pain 249
Jaung-Geng Lin, Kuen-Bao Chen and Yu-Chen Lee

39 Elbow Pain 251
Jaung-Geng Lin, Kuen-Bao Chen and Yu-Chen Lee

40 Wrist Pain 253
Jaung-Geng Lin, Kuen-Bao Chen and Yu-Chen Lee

41 Ankle Pain 255
Jaung-Geng Lin, Kuen-Bao Chen and Yu-Chen Lee

42 Heel Pain 257
Jaung-Geng Lin, Kuen-Bao Chen and Yu-Chen Lee

43 Insomnia 259
Jaung-Geng Lin, Kuen-Bao Chen and Yu-Chen Lee

44 Nausea and Vomiting 261
Jaung-Geng Lin, Kuen-Bao Chen and Yu-Chen Lee

45 Sedation 263
Jaung-Geng Lin, Kuen-Bao Chen and Yu-Chen Lee

46 Dizziness 265
Jaung-Geng Lin, Kuen-Bao Chen and Yu-Chen Lee

Index 267

Contributors

Kuen-Bao Chen, MD, Msc Department of Anesthesiology, China Medical University Hospital, Taichung, Taiwan, Republic of China

Jen-Hwey Chiu, MD, PhD Institute of Traditional Medicine, School of Medicine, National Yang-Ming University; Division of General Surgery, Department of Surgery, Taipei Veterans General Hospital, Peitou, Taipei, Taiwan, Republic of China

Eric Shen-Zen Hsu, MD Pain Management Center, Santa Monica-UCLA Medical Center and Orthopedic Hospital, Santa Monica, California, USA

Annie D. Lee, MD Department of Anesthesiology, University California at Los Angeles, Los Angeles, USA

Tat Leang Lee, MBBS, MMed (Anaesthesia), FANZCA Anaesthesia and Acupuncture Service, National University of Singapore, National University Hospital, Singapore

Yu-Chen Lee, MD Department of Acupuncture, China Medical University Hospital, Taichung, Taiwan, Republic of China

Jaung-Geng Lin, CMD, MD, PhD School of Chinese Medicine, China Medical University, Taichung, Taiwan, Republic of China

Yuan-Chi Lin, MD, MPH Medical Acupuncture Service, Department of Anesthesiology, Perioperative and Pain Medicine, Boston Children's Hospital; Harvard Medical School, Boston, Massachusetts, USA

Francisco Lozano, MD, PhD Medical Acupuncture Specialty, National School of medicine & Homeopathy, National Polytechnic Institute, Ticomán, México D.F., Mexico

Yue-Pang Mok, MD Akron, Ohio, USA

Lynn M. Rusy, MD, FAAMA Department of Anesthesia, Children's Hospital of Wisconsin, Milwaukee, Wisconsin, USA

Yung-Fong Sung, MD, FACA Professor Emeritus, Emory University, School of Medicine, Medical Director Emeritus, Ambulatory Surgical Centers, The Emory Clinic, INC. Emory Health Care, Atlanta, Georgia, USA

Rosalie F. Tassone, MD, MPH Department of Anesthesiology, University of Illinois at Chicago, Chicago, Illinois, USA

Cynthia S. Tung, MD, MPH Medical Acupuncture Service, Department of Anesthesiology, Perioperative and Pain Medicine, Boston Children's Hospital; Harvard Medical School, Boston, Massachusetts, USA

Shu-Ming Wang, MS, MD Anesthesiology and Perioperative Care, University of California, Irvine, Orange, California, USA

Zhen Zheng, BMed, PhD Traditional and Complementary Medicine Research Program, Health Innovations Research Institute & School of Health Sciences, RMIT University, Bundoora, Victoria, Australia

Part I
General Consideration

Chapter 1
History of Acupuncture

Jen-Hwey Chiu

Introduction

Acupuncture, an ancient medical technique of traditional Chinese medicine practiced for over 2,500 years, was first introduced into the US mainstream society in 1971. Among three major indications of the treatment (pain relief, functional adjustment, and immune modulation), acupuncture analgesia (AA) is the most widely used treatment in humans. Thanks to the advances in biochemical and biophysical technology, the mechanisms of AA are elucidated as a consequence of peripheral acupoint stimulation, mobilization of central neural peptides, and triggering of the central inhibitory pathway for modulation of pain sensation. A comprehensive understanding of the origin and history of acupuncture will help Western scientists integrate this ancient technique as a complementary practice into modern medicine.

Definition of Acupuncture

"Acupmoxa" is a hybrid word of "acupuncture" and "moxibustion", which closely resembles the Chinese ideograph for this treatment. Acupuncture involves penetration of skin areas (acupoints) with thin metallic needles, followed by manipulation of the needles, either manually or by electrical stimulation. Moxibustion is a technique in which heat is applied to acupoints through the burning of compressed, powdered herbal materials at the acupoints to be stimulated [1]. Acupuncture or moxibustion, either alone or in combination with each other, can be applied for the treatment of many diseases [2].

J.-H. Chiu (✉)
Institute of Traditional Medicine, School of Medicine, National Yang-Ming University, No. 155, Sec. II, Li-Nong Street, Peitou, Taipei, Taiwan 112, Republic of China
e-mail: chiujh@mailsrv.ym.edu.tw

Division of General Surgery, Department of Surgery, Taipei Veterans General Hospital, Peitou, No. 155, Sec. II, Li-Nong Street, Taipei, Taiwan 112, Republic of China

Origin of Acupuncture

In contrast to Western medicine, which can be traced back to Hippocrates in a clear distinct path, Chinese acupuncture theory was fully developed by the end of second century BC. There is undocumented evidence that the tattoo marks on the Tyrolean Iceman (dated to 3300 BCE) coincide with acupuncture points known to us today. This may date the origin of acupuncture back to time immemorial, and indicate its spread beyond China, or perhaps a spontaneous development in other regions of the world [3]. However, among many old civilizations, such as kingdoms in Africa, Sumer, China, Mesoamerica, and Indus-Ganges, China is the only civilization where acupuncture was well documented 2,000 years ago.

In 1972, documents were discovered in China, written on silk scrolls from the Ma Wang Dui tomb (sealed in 198 BCE). These documents referred to moxibustion, without reference to acupuncture or acupoints, and included 11 lines of channel (meridians). This suggests that the origins of moxibustion and meridians predate those of acupuncture and acupoints [4].

The first document (dated about 100 BCE) to systemically describe acupuncture's use in treating human disorder through the propelling of hypothetic "qi" (vital energy or life force) in the meridians is titled *Ling Shu* (translation: *The Spiritual Pivot*). *Ling Shu* is the second part of an ancient Chinese textbook of medicine with the English title *The Yellow Emperor's Classic of Internal Medicine* (*Nei Jing* in Chinese). The first part of the book, the *Su Wen* (or *Simple Questions* or *Plain Questions* in English), describes the treatment strategy of traditional Chinese medicine. For a thousand years, the principles and logical intension described in *Ling Shu* remain the central dogma of acupuncture treatment.

History of Acupuncture

Before Documentation of Acupuncture

The clan commune period in China began about 100,000 years ago, and lasted until 4,000 years ago. Before the first documentation of acupuncture, or *Ling Shu*, acupuncture instruments are postulated to have been made from sharpened stone called "bian stone," also referred to as "needle stone," or "arrow-headed stone." "Bian" indicates treating disease with stone, and the "bian stone" is an ancient device that was employed for external treatment. Described in chapter 12 of *Su Wen*, bian stones could be found along the seashore, and were the first choice in treating human disorders such as abscesses. Discovered relics of bian stone ranging from 4.5 to 9.1 cm in size provide powerful evidence of acupuncture's origin in eastern China.

1 History of Acupuncture

Table 1.1 Classification and function of the Nine Needles for acupuncture

Types	Length Traditional[a] (100 BCE)	Length Metric (cm)	Functions
Chisel-like needle	1'6"	3.696	Superficial piercing
Round-tipped needle	1'6"	3.696	Massaging acupoints
Chih needle	3'5"	8.085	Knocking or pressing points
Tri-edegd needle	1'6"	3.696	Venipuncture or blood-letting
Pi needle	4'	9.240	Drainage of abscesses
Round-sharp needle	1'6"	3.696	Rapid pricking
Filiform needle	1'6"	3.696	Model for today's needles
Long needle	7'	16.170	Muscle insertion
Large needle	4'	9.240	Joint insertion

[a] Traditional measurement scale: 1'6" = 1 Cun 6 Fen (100 BCE)

Evolution of Acupuncture Needles

The evolution of the acupuncture needle has historically been connected with cultural backgrounds and available local materials. In the Shang Dynasty (1000 BCE), for example, hieroglyphs of acupuncture appeared in inscriptions on bones or shells, but with the development of bronze casting techniques, bronze needles appeared. Upon the introduction and application of iron instruments between 475 BCE and 24 AD, bian stones were replaced by metallic needles, opening a new era for acupuncture practice with ease of handling.

According to the description in *Ling Shu*, there were nine types of metallic needles ("the Nine Needles") at that time, with varying shapes and uses: the chisel-like needle, round-tipped needle, chih needle, tri-edged needle, *pi* (sword-like) needle, round sharp needle, filiform needle, long needle, and large needle. The length and function of the Nine Needles are shown in Table 1.1. In 1308 AD, the figures of "the Nine Needles" were first illustrated in the book *Chi Shen Ba Tuei*, followed by subsequent versions, and again demonstrated in *The Great Compendium of Acupuncture and Moxibustion* (1601) (see Fig. 1.1). Modern needles currently used to achieve pain relief are derived from the filiform needle.

Lineage of Meridian and Acupoint

As mentioned previously, silk scrolls discovered in 198 BCE contain the only evidence of moxibustion and 11 lines of meridian, without any reference to acupuncture or

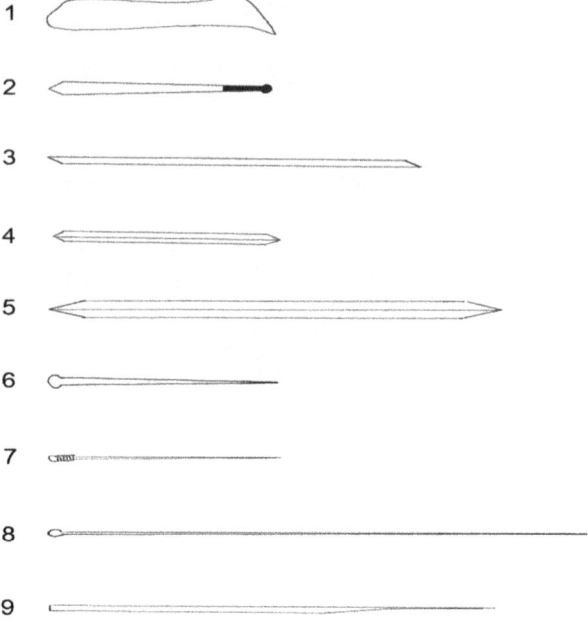

Fig. 1.1 The Nine Needles from "The Great Compendium of Acupuncture and Moxibustion" (1601). They were chisel-like needle (*1*), round-tipped needle (*2*), *chih* needle (*3*), tri-edged needle (*4*), *pi* (sword-like) needle (*5*), round sharp needle (*6*), filiform needle (*7*), long needle (*8*), and large needle (*9*). The needles still currently in use for pain relief are derived from the filiform needle

acupoints [4]. It is reasonable to deduce that the acupoints currently in common use are plotted upon these original meridians. In the time following the discovery of the Ma Wang Dui texts, much literature was produced relating to the development of acupoint localization. One example, *Systematic Classic of Acupuncture and Moxibustion* compiled by Huangfu Mi (256–260), consists of 12 volumes with 128 chapters. It includes 349 acupoints and is one of the most influential works in the history of acupuncture and moxibustion. *Prescriptions for Emergencies* by Ge Hong (265–581) popularized medical knowledge, especially the therapeutic methods of acupuncture and moxibustion. Further modification by acupuncture experts for centuries has resulted in the number of meridians and acupoints increasing to 12 regular and eight extra meridians and 365 points in total, respectively.

By the Tang dynasties (618–907), acupuncture was recognized as a specialized branch of medicine, and those practicing in the field bore the title "Acupuncturist." Supported by the Northern Song government (1026), the book *Illustrated Manual on the Points for Acupuncture and Moxibustion on a New Bronze Figure* describes in detail the locations of acupoints, their related meridians, and includes a supplement to their indications. This publication was followed by the manufacture of two bronze statues designed by Wang Weiyi (1027), depicting the internal organs set inside and the meridians and acupoints engraved on the surface for teaching and examination purposes.

Traditional Concept of Pain Relief by Acupuncture

Although controversy exists concerning the true nature of "meridians," there is consensus that circulation of qi in the meridians is essential for the maintenance of normal body functions. According to the description in *Ling Shu*, there are two hypotheses about the characteristics of meridians: (1) a meridian is a space containing those structures essential for qi transportation and (2) qi is a vital energy, indicating that only live persons can drive the circulation of qi. In traditional Chinese medicine, pain and illness are interpreted as symptoms that occur when the corresponding meridians are blocked (known as the "meridian blocked theory"). Acupuncture treatment can unblock these meridians, thereby reestablishing the flow of qi and relieving the symptoms. These hypotheses, however, have not yet been validated by modern science and technology.

Recent Study on Acupuncture Analgesia

The Role of Endogenous Opioids in Acupuncture Analgesia

In the early 1970s when acupuncture was first introduced to the USA, gate theory and diffuse noxious inhibitory control (DNIC) models were used to explain its effectiveness [5, 6]. Nearly at the same time β-endorphin (1976) was discovered by Li and Chung, amidst a flurry of discoveries in the field of "endogenous opiates," which also included Met-enkephalin, Leu- enkephalin (1975), dynorphin (1979), and more recently, the endomorphin (1997), and were postulated to act as potent analgesic agents [7–10]. The relationship between AA and different kinds of endogenous opiates was then explored in detail. The most well-known group is Han JS's. They postulated that the mechanisms of AA is through peripheral stimulation of acupoints and mediated by mobilization of central neuropeptides [9, 11, 12]. Furthermore, stimulation by different frequencies (2, 15, 100 Hz) on destined points on the skin surface mobilizes different neuropeptides (β-endorphin, enkephalin, dynorphin), bind to the corresponding receptors (μ-opioid receptor, δ-opioid receptor, κ-opioid receptor) and induce analgesic effects, respectively [9, 13].

The Role of Serotonin and the Descending Inhibitory Pathway in Acupuncture Analgesia

Acupuncture-induced analgesic effect is demonstrated not only in humans but also in rabbits and rats. In addition to opioids, other central substances such as 5-hydroxytryptamine (5-HT) [14–17] and spinal orphanin and norepinephrine (NE) are related to AA effect, whereas central cholecystokinin-8 (CCK-8), NE, and orphanin are related to tolerance of AA [18–20].

Evidence for Acupuncture Analgesia

Recent history of AA can be traced back to the late 1950s, when the clinical practice of AA in China was used as a technique to induce analgesic effects during surgery [21]. Evidence (level IV) showing acupuncture's use was reported in 1971, when *New York Times* reporter James Reston wrote about doctors in China using needles to ease his pain after appendectomy [22]. To collect scientific evidence of acupuncture's effectiveness, randomized controlled trials began emerging in 1992. By 2000, 12 articles on the subject had been published, increasing to 113 by the end of 2009 [23].

Two consensus meetings were held for acupuncture research, which contributed to efficacy exploration of this ancient technique, despite some skeptical critiques [24–26]. The first of these meetings, entitled "NIH Consensus Development Conference on Acupuncture," was held in 1997 in Bethesda, MD [27]. A World Health Organization report and a National Institutes of Health consensus conference each provided long lists of indications for which acupuncture was allegedly of proven benefit. The second "NIH Consensus Development Conference on Acupuncture," held in 2007, summarized not only AA but also the modulation of visceral functions and anti-inflammation as acupuncture indications [28].

There is still work to be done to improve scientific AA research. During the past few decades, researchers have addressed their greatest methodological challenge, placebo needling. Cochrane's recent reviews of acupuncture for the treatment of any type of pain suggest that acupuncture is effective for some, but not all, types of pain [29]. In summary, areas of consensus and controversy exist, and large scale, well-designed clinical trials are still needed to reveal the mysteries of AA with results that pass muster with scientists [26, 30, 31].

fMRI Study on Acupuncture Analgesia

In addition to the discovery of biochemical substances, such as endogenous neuropeptides, advancements in technology have contributed to the advancement of acupuncture research as well. Functional magnetic resonance imaging (fMRI) allows researchers to obtain visualization of the brain at the moment of sensory stimulation.

The first acupuncture research study employing magnetic resonance imaging was reported in 1998. It may prove to be a landmark study, despite having been withdrawn by the authors in 2006 [32]. Since the start of the current millennium, much effort has been devoted to acupuncture-related fMRI or positron emission tomography (PET) studies. The accumulating evidence suggests that acupuncture modulates many distributed cortical and subcortical brain areas [33–37]. These brain areas support endogenous antinociceptive mechanisms and part of the pain neuromatrix, and may contribute to the therapeutic effect of acupuncture by shifting the autonomic nervous system balance and altering the affective and cognitive dimensions of pain processing [38, 39]. There is also evidence, both in animals and in

1 History of Acupuncture

Table 1.2 Chronicle of AA

Year	Events related to AA
~5000 BCE	Sharpened stones as tools of acupuncture [2]
3300 BCE	Tattoo marks on the Tyrolean Iceman [3]
198 BCE	Silk scrolls (origin of moxibustion) [4]
100 BCE	*The Yellow Emperor's Classic of Internal Medicine*, 1st document (Ling Shu) describing AA [2]
1950s	AA developed in China [21]
1965	Gate theory for AA [5]
1971	Introduction of AA into USA [22]
1975	Discovery of enkephalin [9]
1976	Discovery of endorphin [7, 8]
1979	Discovery of dynorphin [9], non-endorphin system for AA [14], DNIC theory for AA [6]
1986	Cholecystokinin 8 as a mediator for AA tolerance [18]
1997	Discovery of endomorphin [10], 1st NIH consensus meeting on acupuncture [27]
1998	1st fMRI study for AA studies [32]
2007	2nd NIH consensus meeting on acupuncture [28]

AA acupuncture analgesia, *DNIC* diffuse noxious inhibitory control, *NIH* National Institute of Health, *fMRI* functional magnetic resonance imaging

humans, that sham electroacupuncture (EA) and real EA both activated the reported distributed pain neuromatrix. Real EA, however, elicited significantly higher activation over the hypothalamus and primary somatosensory–motor cortex than sham EA, as well as deactivation over the rostral segment of anterior cingulate cortex. This may explain the relative acupuncture specificity in clinical aspect [40–42].

Conclusion

There is an increasing trend in people outside Asia using acupuncture as a complementary treatment for their disorders. For the past four decades, extensive studies of both the basic and clinical aspects have rigorously explored the efficacy and mechanisms of AA. Becoming familiar with the recent history of AA (see Table 1.2) provides a better understanding of the benefits of integrating the practice into current, western, medical pain management.

References

1. The Academy of Traditional Chinese Medicine. An outline of Chinese acupuncture. Peking: Foreign Languages Press; 1975.
2. Cheng XN, editor. Chinese acupuncture and moxibustion. Beijing: Foreign Languages Press; 1987.
3. Dorfer L, Moser M, Bahr F, et al. A medical report from the stone age? Lancet. 1999;354(9183):1023–5.
4. Chen Y. Silk scrolls: earliest literature of meridian doctrine in ancient China. Acupunct Electrother Res. 1997;22(3–4):175–89.
5. Melzack R, Wall PD. Pain mechanisms: a new theory. Science. 1965;150(699):971–9.
6. Le Bars D, Dickenson AH, Besson JM. Diffuse noxious inhibitory controls (DNIC). I. Effects on dorsal horn convergent neurones in the rat. Pain 1979;6(3):283–304.
7. Li CH, Chung D. Isolation and structure of an untriakontapeptide with opiate activity from camel pituitary glands. Proc Natl Acad Sci U S A. 1976;73(4):1145–8.
8. Loh HH, Tseng LF, Wei E, et al. β-Endorphin is a potent analgesic agent. Proc Natl Acad Sci U S A. 1976;73(8):2895–8.
9. Han JS. Acupuncture and endorphins. Neurosci Lett. 2004;361(1–3):258–61.
10. Zadina JE, Hackler L, Ge LJ, et al. A potent and selective endogenous agonist for the m-opiate receptor. Nature. 1997;386(6624):499–502.
11. Chen XH, Han JS. Analgesia induced by electroacupuncture of different frequencies is mediated by different types of opioid receptors: another cross-tolerance study. Behav Brain Res. 1992;47(2):143–9.
12. Han JS. Acupuncture analgesia: areas of consensus and controversy. Pain. 2011;152(3 Suppl):S41–8.
13. Taguchi R, Taguchi T, Kitakoji H. Involvement of peripheral opioid receptors in electroacupuncture analgesia for carrageenan-induced hyperalgesia. Brain Res. 2010;1355:97–103.
14. Cheng RS, Pomeranz B. Electroacupuncture analgesia could be mediated by at least two pain-relieving mechanisms; endorphin and non-endorphin systems. Life Sci. 1979;25(23):1957–62.
15. Tsai HY, Lin JG, Inoki R. Further evidence for possible analgesic mechanism of electroacupuncture: effects on neuropeptides and serotonergic neurons in rat spinal cord. Jpn J Pharmacol. 1989;49(2):181–5.
16. Baek YH, Choi DY, Yang HI, et al. Analgesic effect of electroacupuncture on inflammatory pain in the rat model of collagen-induced arthritis: mediation by cholinergic and serotonergic receptors. Brain Res. 2005;1057(1–2):181–5.
17. Lin JG, Chen WL. Acupuncture analgesia: a review of its mechanisms of actions. Am J Chin Med. 2008;36(4):635–45.
18. Han JS, Ding XZ, Fan SG. Cholecystokinin octapeptide (CCK-8): antagonism to electroacupuncture analgesia and a possible role in electroacupuncture tolerance. Pain. 1986;27(1):101–15.
19. Han JS. Cholecystokinin octapeptide (CCK-8): a negative feedback control mechanism for opioid analgesia. Prog Brain Res. 1995;105:263–71.
20. Tian JH, Xu W, Fang Y, et al. Antagonistic effect of orphanin FQ on morphine analgesia in rat brain. Sheng Li Xue Bao. 1997;49(3):333–8.
21. Wu GC. Acupuncture anesthesia in China: retrospect and prospect. Chin J Integr Med. 2007;13(3):163–5.
22. Reston J. Now, about my operation in Peking; now, let me tell you about my appendectomy in Peking. The New York Times. 26 July 1971.
23. Han JS, Ho YS. Global trends and performances of acupuncture research. Neurosci Biobehav Rev. 2011;35(3):680–7.
24. Skrabanek P. Acupuncture and the age of unreason. Lancet. 1984;1(8387):1169–71.
25. Sampson WI. Acupuncture: the position paper of the National Council Against Health Fraud. Clin J Pain. 1991;7:162–6.

26. Ernst E. The recent history of acupuncture. Am J Med. 2008;121(12):1027–8.
27. NIH Consensus Conference. Acupuncture. JAMA. 1998;280:1518–24.
28. Napadow V, Ahn A, Longhurst J, et al. The status and future of acupuncture mechanism research. J Altern Complement Med. 2008;14(7):861–9.
29. Lee MS, Ernst E. Acupuncture for pain: an overview of Cochrane reviews. Chin J Integr Med. 2011;17(3):187–9.
30. Mann F. Reinventing acupuncture. Oxford: Butterworth Heinemann; 1992.
31. Ulett G. Beyond Yin and Yang: how acupuncture really works. St. Louis: Warren H Green; 1992.
32. Cho ZH, Chung SC, Lee HJ, et al. Retraction. New findings of the correlation between acupoints and corresponding brain cortices using functional MRI. Proc Natl Acad Sci U S A. 2006;103(27):10527.
33. Wu MT, Hsieh JC, Xiong J, et al. Central nervous pathway for acupuncture stimulation: localization of processing with functional MR imaging of the brain—preliminary experience. Radiology. 1999;212(1):133–41.
34. Hsieh JC, Tu CH, Chen FP, et al. Activation of the hypothalamus characterizes the acupuncture stimulation at the analgesic point in human: a positron emission tomography study. Neurosci Lett. 2001;307(2):105–8.
35. Hui KK, Marina O, Liu J, et al. Acupuncture, the limbic system, and the anticorrelated networks of the brain. Auton Neurosci. 2010;157(1–2):81–90.
36. Napadow V, Dhond R, Park K, et al. Time-variant fMRI activity in the brainstem and higher structures in response to acupuncture. Neuroimage. 2009;47(1):289–301.
37. Fang J, Jin Z, Wang Y, et al. The salient characteristics of the central effects of acupuncture needling: limbic-paralimbic-neocortical network modulation. Hum Brain Mapp. 2009;30(4):1196–206.
38. Fields HL, Basbaum AI. Central nervous system mechanisms of pain modulation. In: Wall PD, Melzack R, editors. Textbook of pain. Edinburgh: Churchill Livingstone; 1999. pp. 309–29.
39. Peets JM, Pomeranz B. CXBK mice deficient in opiate receptors show poor electroacupuncture analgesia. Nature. 1978;273(5664):675–6.
40. Chiu JH, Chung MS, Cheng HC, et al. Different central manifestations in response to electroacupuncture at analgesic and nonanalgesic acupoints in rats: a manganese-enhanced functional magnetic resonance imaging study. Can J Vet Res. 2003;67(2):94–101.
41. Chiu JH, Cheng HC, Tai CH, et al. Electroacupuncture-induced neural activation detected by use of manganese-enhanced functional magnetic resonance imaging in rabbits. Am J Vet Res. 2001;62(2):178–82.
42. Wu MT, Sheen JM, Chuang KH, et al. Neuronal specificity of acupuncture response: a fMRI study with electroacupuncture. Neuroimage. 2002;16(4):1028–37.

Chapter 2
Basic Theories of Traditional Chinese Medicine

Francisco Lozano

Introduction

Traditional Chinese medicine (TCM) is a unique, complete medical system arising from a living tradition of literate scholarship that spans at least 2,000 years. Well structured and resting upon a solid, coherent theoretical basis, TCM provides an integral framework for understanding, interpreting, and organizing interventions in the human health-disease process. Over the course of its long history, TCM in various forms has been the main form of health care in China and many other countries in Asia. Its theories and techniques are studied and practiced alongside Western biomedicine in countries such as Japan, Vietnam, Singapore, Taiwan, and mainland China, and it has become one of the main forms of alternative medicine in North America and Europe.

TCM views the human being as standing in intimate relation to its natural environment. In fact, this relationship is considered a key element in the health of the individual. Disease is understood to be a deviation from natural conditions, which correspond with changes in the natural environment. TCM thus describes diseases as being caused by wind, cold, dampness, heat, and so on, while the internal functions of the body are grouped together according to perceived systemic relationships. What these descriptions point to are clusters of related phenomena in the body, which occur together and can be treated with specific interventions, i.e., acupuncture, herbal therapy, and so on.

The importance of these theories for the application of acupuncture and herbal therapy cannot be underrated. Unlike Western biomedicine, which focuses on structural changes in the body and alterations in the chemical composition of blood and other tissues, the emphasis of TCM theory is in alterations of function. In order to manifest the full therapeutic potential of TCM, the patients and their conditions

F. Lozano (✉)
Medical Acupuncture Specialty, National School of Medicine & Homeopathy, National Polytechnic Institute, Guillermo Massieu Helguera Num. 239, Fraccionamiento la Escalera, Ticomán, México D.F., Mexico
e-mail: lozanof57@gmail.com

Fig. 2.1 Taiji diagram (Tai Ji Tu). The classic yin and yang diagram

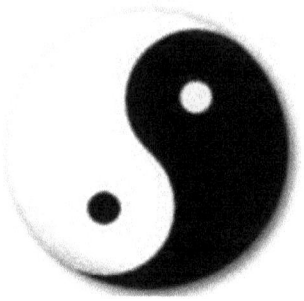

need to be analyzed through the lens of this system. In our experience, this not only optimizes the applicability of TCM-based therapies, such as acupuncture and herbal medicine, but also complements the highly specific approach of Western biomedicine, thereby providing superior health care and optimal clinical results.

Basic Theories of Traditional Chinese Medicine

TCM theory in its present form arose from the naturalistic philosophies of ancient China, influenced and expanded upon by the accumulated clinical experience of generations of literate scholar practitioners. It is because of this cultural context that TCM theory can at times seem abstruse or outdated. However, it represents a complete, integrated method of interpreting human physiology and responding to pathological changes in the body [1].

The most important concepts taken from ancient Chinese naturalistic philosophy in TCM are those of *qi*, *yinyang*, and the five phases (*wuxing*). Theoretical concepts specific to TCM include the doctrine of *zheng ti guang nian*, the concepts of the viscera and bowels (*zangfu xue shuo*), channels and networks (*jingluo*), body substances (*qi*, blood, essence and body fluids *qi xue jing jinye*); and pathogenic agents (*bing yin*). These theories, together with the methodologies of the four (diagnostic) methods (*si zhen*) and pattern discrimination (*bian zheng*) comprise the theoretical framework of TCM. Each of the therapeutic tools of TCM, including acupuncture and moxibustion (*zhenjiu*), Chinese herbology (*zhongyao fang*), and Chinese therapeutic massage (*zhongyi tuina*) rest upon this theoretical basis [2–7].

Yinyang Theory (yinyang xue shuo)

Yinyang theory expresses a universal standard of quality that describes two complementary, opposite aspects of an indivisible whole (Fig. 2.1). It is used to describe function and relationship of these aspects as part of a continuous process of transformation and change in the universe. Applied to medicine, *yinyang* theory is used to compare and contrast, and thus differentiate, physiological and pathological phenomena.

Yin is associated to qualities such as cold, rest, responsiveness, passivity, darkness, structure, the interior, downward and inward motion, and decrease. By contrast, *yang* is associated with heat, stimulation, movement, activity, light, the exterior, upward and outward motion, and increase. It is important to observe that these aspects occur only in relation to each other (i.e., cold can be defined only by the knowledge of heat, darkness by the presence or absence of light, and so on). In medicine, *yinyang* theory would be applied to opposites such as structure (*yin*) and function (*yang*), the lower body (*yin*) in relation to the upper body (*yang*); however, the concepts of *yinyang* are never absolute. They are applied to given objects in order to express their relation to other objects, actions, or processes.

Yinyang theory has four fundamental characteristics, known as the four relations of *yinyang*:

1. Opposition
2. Interdependence, interdivisibility, and relativity
3. Inter-consuming-supporting
4. Intertransforming

Opposition

As previously mentioned, *yinyang* theory describes a universal qualitative standard. One of the key aspects of this is that the *yin* aspect of something exists only in opposition to its *yang* aspect. Heaven and earth, sun and moon, night and day, male and female, up and down, inside and outside, and quiescence and movement are manifestations of a duality intrinsic to the universe. Water is cold and fire is hot, and water flows downward while fire tends to rise. Therefore, water is *yin* and fire is *yang*. Similarly, day is *yang* and night is *yin*, high is *yang* and low is *yin,* matter is *yin* and energy is *yang*, and the passive element is *yin* and the active element is *yang*.

In terms of medicine, the upper body is *yang* in relation to the lower body, which is *yin*. However, the anterior side of the body is *yin* while the posterior side is *yang*. The medial aspect of the extremities is *yin* while the lateral aspect is *yang*. As a whole, the interior of the body is *yin* while the exterior is *yang*. Within the interior of the body, the *zang* organs (sometimes called "viscera"), considered "solid" and in charge of storage, are *yin*, whereas the *fu* organs (sometimes referred to as "bowels") are held to be "hollow" and in charge of discharging their contents, and thus are *yang*. Diseases that manifest signs and symptoms associated with heat and excessive metabolic activity are *yang*, whereas diseases that display cold signs and a decrease in activity are *yin*. Rapid, replete, forceful pulses are *yang*, whereas slow, vacuous, and forceless are *yin*. Medicinal substances are classified as hot or warm (*yang*) and cool or cold (*yin*). As previously mentioned, overall *yin* refers to structure and form in the body, as opposed to function and metabolic activity, which are *yang* (Table 2.1).

Table 2.1 Basic *yinyang* correspondences used in TCM

Yin	*Yang*
Water	Fire
Cold	Hot
Interior	Exterior
Slow	Rapid
Passivity	Activity
Quiescence	Movement
Lower position or downward direction	Upper position or upward direction
Interior position or inward direction	Exterior position or outward direction
Dimness	Brightness
Inhibition	Excitation
Weakness	Strength
Hypoactivity	Hyperactivity
Structure	Function
Internal organs	Body surface
Zang organs	*Fu* organs
Lower body, below the waist	Upper body, above the waist
Anterior region	Posterior region
Medial aspect of the limbs	Lateral aspect of the limbs
Right side	Left side
Qi	Blood

Interdependence

Yin and *yang* define aspects of a whole, and therefore, they depend on each other. The whole is defined by the existence of the two opposing aspects. "Cold" cannot be defined without "heat," "above" is meaningless without "below," and "exterior" and "interior" mutually define each other. This is all in relation to a whole that contains these two parts.

In medicine, the clearest example of *yinyang* interdependence is the relationship between structure and function. Structure (or form) pertains to *yin*, and function to *yang*. Together, they are complementary aspects of the whole that is the living body. Sufficient substance (structure) in the form of body fluids, healthy tissue, etc., allows for normal function. In turn, only when the functional processes are in good condition can the essential substances be appropriately replenished. The balance between structure and function is the basis for healthy physiological activity.

Interdivisibility and Relativity Because *yinyang* are aspects of the whole, no object, phenomenon, event, or situation can ever be labeled as purely or wholly *yin* or *yang*. Phenomena in the universe have *yin* and *yang* aspects, depending on the viewpoint of analysis. For example, day is considered *yang* when compared with night, but the early hours of the day (before noon) are *yang* when compared with the hours after noon, which are *yin*. In Chinese thought, it is said that the morning is *yang* within *yang*, and the afternoon is *yin* within *yang*. These hierarchies of *yin* and *yang* can be extended ad infinitum, as each separate phenomenon can be divided into its *yin* and *yang* aspect.

Inter-consuming-supporting

In *yinyang* theory, a gain, growth, or advance of one aspect of the whole means a loss, decline, or retreat of the other (this is sometimes referred to as "the waxing and waning" of *yin* and *yang*). Under normal conditions, this consumption/support occurs within limits. In terms of physiology, it could be likened to homeostasis. Exceeding these limits results in dysfunction and disease, but here, too, we may see the consumption of one by the other. A *yang* disorder, with an excess of metabolic activity, will gradually consume the resources (*yin*) of the body. Conversely, cold congelation or advanced age (*yin*) can bring about a drastic reduction of body function (*yang*). In terms of pathology, all diseases can be thought of as pertaining to one of four imbalances along these lines: excess of *yang*, excess of *yin*, deficiency of *yang*, or deficiency of *yin*.

Intertransformation

This back and forth between *yin* and *yang* implies a characteristic of constant motion and transformation, which is observed in the world. *Yin* transforms into *yang*, and *yang* in turn evolves into *yin*. The *yang* day transforms into the *yin* night, just like shadows moving across the face of a mountain as the sun travels across the horizon.

In terms of medicine, the intertransformation of *yinyang* can be said to occur in two ways: harmoniously, as in the natural course of development, growth, aging, and death, and deviating from the norm, as in response to drastic environmental changes or internal imbalance. Normally, *yin* and *yang* follow each other naturally, and this constant transformation is the source of life as we observe it. We could call this smooth, successive process as "health." In disease, this process is disrupted and *yin* and *yang* are out of balance—an excess of one, which automatically presupposes a deficiency of the other. This can continue to the point where intertransformation occurs, but as a progression of disease. Chinese medical thought holds that "when the exuberance of *yin* reaches and extreme, it will transform into *yang*; when heat blazes, it transforms into cold." This is observable when, for example, a very high fever (which would be a *yang* disorder) causes shock with hypothermia, loss of consciousness, etc. (*yin* symptoms).

Application in Traditional Chinese Medicine

Yinyang theory permeates every aspect of TCM. As can be seen from the examples given above, it is used as a framework to understand anatomy, physiology, pathology, diagnosis, and treatment. Its importance cannot be overrated.

Five-Phase (wuxing) Theory

Five-phase theory establishes a system of correspondences that groups phenomena in the universe into five categories. These categories represent tendencies of movement and transformation in the universe, and are associated with the natural phenomena of wood (*mu*), fire (*huo*), earth (*tu*), metal (*jin*), and water (*shui*). Clear, constant relationships between them are used to explain changes in nature.

Five-Phase Categorization

Each of the phases represents a category of related functions and qualities. Wood is associated with the season of spring, sprouting, early growth, awakening, morning, childhood, and the penetrating, powerful impetus of new life, anger, and wind. Fire is associated with summer. It represents a maximum state of activity, flourishing, exuberant growth, outward motion, high noon, and the expansive movement of happiness and open flame. Earth is associated with the long summer (or the transition between seasons). It signals balance and equilibrium, the early afternoon, nourishment, abundance, the quiet of pensiveness and worry, and dampness. Metal is associated with the autumn season, declining function, a movement toward crystallization and shedding that is not needed, dusk, clarity and sadness, and dry weather. Water is associated with winter. It expresses a state of downward motion, accumulation, rest, nighttime, and the development of new potential, the concentration of willpower and fear, and the cold.

Five phase correspondences permeate all aspects of classical thought in China. The five-way categorization is applied to colors, sounds, odors, flavors, emotions, animals, the planets, and ultimately everything in the universe (see Table 2.2).

Relationships Between the Five Phases

The five phases succeed each other in cycles, acting upon each other in fixed ways. Two cyclical relationships are held to exist among the five phases: an engendering (*sheng*) cycle and a controlling (*ke*) cycle. Both of these cycles are deemed to be natural and necessary. Without engenderment, there is no life; without control, things become excessive.

2 Basic Theories of Traditional Chinese Medicine

Table 2.2 Five-phase correspondences

	Wood	Fire	Earth	Metal	Water
Direction	East	South	Center	West	North
Season	Spring	Summer	Late summer	Fall	Winter
Climate	Wind	Heat	Dampness	Dryness	Cold
Planet	Jupiter	Mars	Saturn	Venus	Mercury
Number	3+5=8	2+5=7	5	4+5=9	1+5=6
Meat	Chicken	Goat	Beef	Horse	Pork
Cereal	Wheat	Millet	Sorghum	Rice	Beans (soy)
Sound	Jiao	Zheng	Gong	Shang	Yu
Musical note	C	D	E	G	A
Color	Green	Red	Yellow	White	Black
Taste	Bitter	Acid	Sweet	Pungent	Salt
Smell	Uremic	Burnt	Scented	Cool	Putrid
Organ	Liver	Heart	Spleen	Lung	Kidney
Viscera	Urinary bladder	Small intestine	Stomach	Large intestine	Bladder
Senses organ	Eyes	Tongue	Mouth	Nose	Ear
Tissue	Tendons	Vessels	Muscles	Skin	Bones
Bodily sounds	Hu (sigh)	Laugh	Singing	Crying	Moan
Virtues	Benevolence	Courtesy	Fidelity	Justice	Knowledge
Emotion	Anger	Joy	Worry	Melancholy	Fear
Spiritual activity[a]	*Hun*	*Shen*	*Yi*	*Po*	*Zhi*
Bodily region	Neck, nape	Thoracocostal	Spine	Escapulodorsal	Lumbar

[a] Hun corresponds to a number of actions equivalent to unconscious activity, but it is also related to deep sleep, etc. Shen is the mental activity, the substrate of thought. Yi is the thought, the ability to generate ideas. Po is the vegetative activity, automatism, etc. Zhi is the will, perseverance, etc.

Engendering Cycle This is the cycle whereby the phases are believed to proceed in order to generate each other in an orderly sequence. The natural action or movement of one phase fosters the growth or waxing of the next, thus wood engenders fire, fire engenders earth, earth engenders metal, metal engenders water, and water engenders wood. This cycle is also known as the "Mother-Son" relationship, with the engendering phase acting as "mother" to the next (the "son").

Controlling Cycle This cycle follows the sequence in which the phases suppress, control, or inhibit each other. In this sequence, wood controls earth, earth controls water, water controls fire, fire controls metal, and metal controls wood.

Fig. 2.2 The five phases (engendering and controlling cycles)

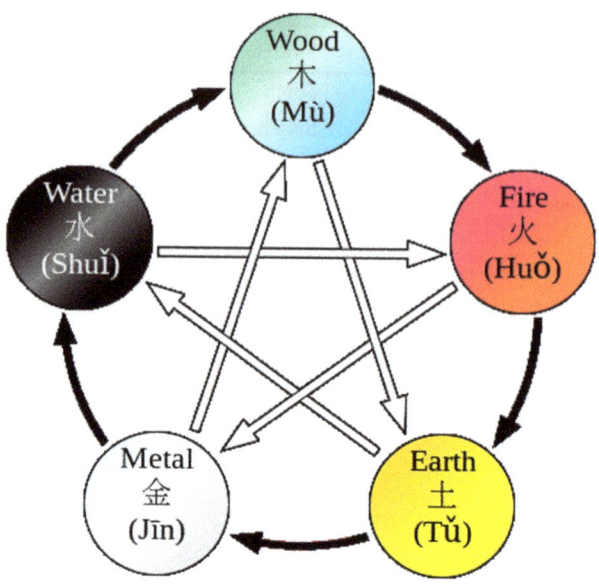

Thus, all phases stand in relationship to the others in one of the four ways: engendering, being engendered, controlling, and being controlled. It follows that the state of one phase in the system is always dependent on the condition of the others. If viewed as aspects of an organic whole, the actions of control and engenderment exerted by each of the phases add up to maintain a dynamic balance (Fig. 2.2).

Five-Phase Theory in Traditional Chinese Medicine

As can be seen from Table 2.2, five-phase correspondences exist in TCM as well. The viscera (*zang*) and bowels (*fu*), along with the acupuncture channels, are classified in this system. Five-phase theory is also used to interpret the physiology and pathology of the human body in relation to the natural environment. It is likewise applied to etiology, diagnosis, treatment, and prognosis.

The main five-phase correspondences used in TCM are those of the *zang* organs: wood is attributed to the liver, which regulates free flow of *qi*; fire is attributed to the heart, which promotes the warming of the whole body; earth is attributed to the spleen, which is in charge of the transportation and transformation of food; metal is attributed to the lung, which promotes the descending of *qi*; and water is attributed to the kidney, which is responsible for the storage of essence and regulating body fluids. The basic engendering and controlling relationships of the five phases are interpreted as follows in physiology:

Engendering Cycle

- Wood engenders fire: the liver stores blood and supplements the blood to be regulated by the heart.
- Fire engenders earth: the heart provides warmth, which is indispensable for the spleen to function.
- Earth engenders metal: the spleen transforms and transports the essential nutrients and sends them up to replenish the lung and support its activity.
- Metal engenders water: the lung, with its clearing and descending functions, sends down *yin* fluids to the kidneys.
- Water engenders wood: Kidney essence nourishes liver blood.

Controlling Cycle

- Wood controls earth: The liver's dredging effect prevents spleen *qi* from becoming stagnant.
- Fire controls metal: The upward and outward movement of heart fire prevents lung *qi* from descending excessively.
- Earth controls water: The action of transportation of the spleen prevents the fluids controlled by the kidney from overflowing.
- Metal controls wood: The clearing and descending action of the lung counteracts the ascent of liver *qi*.
- Water controls fire: Kidney *yin* flows upward to nourish heart *yin*, thus restricting heart *yang*.

Five-Phase Theory in Disease Causation

The engendering and controlling cycles of the five phases are used to explain disease causation, mainly through the "Mother-Son" relationship. In addition, a condition of excess or deficiency in one of the organs can affect other organs by altering the relationships of engenderment and control (see later).

Disease Causation Through the "Mother-Son" Relationship

- Disease of the Mother affecting the Son: If the Mother becomes deficient, it will be unable to nourish the Son, and will eventually cause a deficiency of the Son. For example, a deficiency of the kidney essence (water) will negatively impact the production of liver blood (wood), gradually inducing a condition of liver deficiency. Conversely, if the Mother is affected by an excess condition, this may cause the Son to become excessive as well. For example, if liver fire (wood) flares upward, it will cause heart fire (fire) to become exuberant, leading to an overabundance of fire in the liver and heart.
- Disease of the Son affecting the Mother: In most cases, a disease of the Son will induce a deficiency of the Mother. For example, a deficiency of kidney *yin* can induce a deficiency of lung *yin*, leading to deficiency of both organs. This is explained as due to the increased supply from the Mother to the deficient Son eventually exhausting the resources of the Mother.

Disease Causation Through Deficiency or Excess of an Organ

- Deficiency of one of the organs can induce any of the following scenarios:
  - Deficiency of the Son due to reduction of nourishment
  - Deficiency of the Mother due to increased demand for nourishment
  - Overcontrolling from its controller, which would aggravate the deficiency
  - Counter-domination by its controlled organ
- Excess of one of the organs can result in any of the following:
  - Excess of the Son
  - Excess of the Mother
  - Over-controlling of its controlled organ, causing debilitation of the latter
  - Counter-domination of its controlling organ, causing its debilitation

Five Phases in Diagnosis and Analysis of Symptoms

It is important to point out that although five-phase correspondences exist for many diagnostic signs (see Table 2.2), in actual clinical practice, these findings need to be correlated to the entire diagnostic picture developed through the use of the four methods. In all cases, TCM needs to correlate a large amount of concurrent data in order to arrive at a diagnosis and, in this context, the actual relevance or meaning of any one sign or symptom may vary when analyzed in relation to the whole.

That being said, certain signs, such as facial complexion, odor, tone of voice, etc., can be used as indicators of disease or pathology affecting the corresponding viscus per five-phase theory, or the associated Mother-organ or Son-organ. This can, in some cases, be used also to construct an entire therapeutic strategy according to the five-phase engendering and controlling cycles, as will be explained in the next section.

Five Phases in Therapeutics

As we have seen, disease of one viscus may affect other viscera according to the engendering and controlling cycles of the five phases. Therefore, certain pathological conditions are deemed to be the result of an imbalance between two or more viscera, as opposed to only the imbalance of one viscus. This is borne out in clinical practice by the clusters of associated symptoms and signs that often occur together, and which are associated with specific conditions in TCM diagnostic theory.

It follows that treatment should focus on regulating these relationships. In some cases, this means to treat the affected organ/phase system. However, a therapeutic strategy using the Mother-Son relationship is considered very effective. As the adage goes, "In case of deficiency, tonify the Mother; in case of excess, drain the Son." There are common examples of this in clinical practice (such as tonifying kidney *yin* in order to help resolve a deficiency of liver blood), but the majority of five-phase-based treatment strategies used in modern TCM practice involve the use of a special group of acupuncture points known as the transport-*shu* points.

Table 2.3 The five transport-*shu* points of the *yang* channels

	Jing-Well (metal)	Ying-Spring (water)	Shu-Stream (wood)	Jing-River (fire)	He-Sea (earth)
Gallbladder (wood)	Zuqiaoyin GB 44	Xiaxi GB 43	Zulinqi GB 41	Yangfu GB 38	Yanglingquan GB 34
Small intestine (fire)	Shaoze SI 1	Qiangu SI 2	Houxi SI 3	Yanggu SI 5	Xiaohai SI 8
Sanjiao (fire)	Guanchong SJ 1	Yemen SJ 2	Zhongzhu SJ 3	Zhigou SJ 6	Tianjing SJ 10
Stomach (earth)	Lidui ST 45	Neiting ST 44	Xiangu ST 43	Jiexi ST 41	Zusanli ST 36
Large intestine (metal)	Shangyang LI 1	Erjian LI 2	Sanjian LI 3	Yangxi LI 5	Quchi LI 11
Bladder (water)	Zhiyin BL 67	Zutonggu BL 66	Shugu BL 65	Kunlun BL 60	Weizhong BL 40

Each of the acupuncture channels is associated with either a viscus or a bowel, and with one of the five phases. In addition, each of the channels has five points, located in its most distal locations, which are associated with the five phases (Tables 2.3 and 2.4). Treatment using the transport-*shu* points follows the Mother-Son law. The point associated with the Mother of the affected viscus or bowel is tonified in cases of deficiency, or the point associated with the Son is drained in case of excess (Table 2.5). Sometimes, the corresponding point on the Mother-channel or Son-channel is also used (see Tables 2.6 and 2.7).

Theory of the Viscera and Bowels (Zangfu)

Traditional Chinese medical theory describes physiology as a system of functional spheres of influence, known as the *zangfu*. Loosely correlated to the anatomical structures described by Western biomedicine, the "organs" of Chinese medicine interact with one another, and with inputs from the exterior, in predictable, organized ways that constitute the normal activity of the system. Changes and deviations in *zangfu* function can be observed from exterior manifestations, which constitute patterns of disharmony, i.e., disease. At the core of the system are the five *zang* (viscera): lung, heart, liver, spleen, and kidney. All of the other tissues of the body, including sense organs, connective tissues, fluids, excretions, and the six *fu* (bowels: large intestine, small intestine, gallbladder, stomach, bladder, and the *Sanjiao*) are seen as subordinated to the *zang*, which thus represent entire systems of related function. These organ systems are at the core of TCM practice. Diagnosis and treatment all refer there and are ultimately directed toward one or more of the *zangfu* [8].

Table 2.4 The five transport-*shu* points of the *yin* channels

	Jing-Well (wood)	Ying-Spring (fire)	Shu-Stream (earth)	Jing-River (metal)	He-Sea (water)
Liver (wood)	Dadun LR 1	Xingjian LR 2	Taichong LR 3	Zhongfeng LR 4	Ququan LR 8
Heart (fire)	Shaochong HT 9	Shaofu HT 8	Shenmen HT 7	Lingdao HT 4	Shaohai HT 3
Pericardium (fire)	Zhongchong PC 9	Laogong PC 8	Daling PC 7	Jianshi PC 5	Quze PC 3
Spleen (earth)	Yinbai SP 1	Dadu SP 2	Taibai SP 3	Shangqiu SP 5	Yinlingquan SP 9
Lung (metal)	Shaoshang LU 11	Yuji LU 10	Taiyuan LU 9	Jingqu LU 8	Chize LU 5
Kidney (water)	Yongquan KI 1	Rangu KI 2	Taixi KI 3	Fuliu KI 7	Yingu KI 10

Table 2.5 "Mother-Son" points of the 12 regular channels

Channel	Mother point (for tonification)	Son point (for dispersion)
Liver (wood)	Ququan (LR 8) (water)	Xingjian (LR 2) (fire)
Heart (fire)	Shaochong (HT 9) (wood)	Shenmen (HT 7) (earth)
Pericardium (fire)	Zhongchong (PC 9) (wood)	Daling (PC 7) (earth)
Spleen (earth)	Dadu (SP 2) (fire)	Shangqiu (SP 5) (metal)
Lung (metal)	Taiyuan (LU 9) (earth)	Chize (LU 5) (water)
Kidney (water)	Fuliu (KI 7) (metal)	Yongquan (KI 1) (wood)
Gallbladder (wood)	Xiaxi (GB 43) (water)	Yangfu (GB 38) (fire)
Small Intestine (fire)	Houxi (SI 3) (wood)	Xiaohai (SI 8) (earth)
Sanjiao (fire)	Zhongzhu (SJ 3) (wood)	Tianjing (SJ 10) (earth)
Stomach (earth)	Jiexi (ST 41) (fire)	Lidui (ST 45) (metal)
Large Intestine (metal)	Quchi (LI 11) (earth)	Erjian (LI 2) (water)
Urinary Bladder (water)	Zhiyin (UB 67) (metal)	Shugu (UB 65) (wood)

As previously explained (see Sect. Five Phase), the theory of the five phases assigns related phenomena into categories that express their "energetic" quality, or movement. These correspondences are used within *zangfu* theory to assign each organ a tissue, a sense organ, an "outgrowth" (usually refers to the accessory structures of the skin), a bodily secretion, a color, a flavor, and so on. These correspondences are then used in diagnosis to trace a given disease manifestation back to the affected organ system(s), and in treatment to select acupuncture points, medicinal substances, and other therapeutic tools to affect the condition from an organic, holistic perspective. Each of the organ systems, their correspondences, and areas of influence, will be discussed next [7–11].

Table 2.6 "Mother-Son" point combinations for deficiency and excess conditions of the *yin* channels

Channel	Condition	Affected channel ("Mother or Son Points")	"Mother-Son Channel" (element points)
Lung (metal)	Deficiency	*Taiyuan* LU 9, earth of the metal channel	*Taibai* SP 3, earth of the earth channel
	Excess	*Chize* LU 5, water of the metal channel	*Yingu* KI 10, water of the water channel
Heart (fire)	Deficiency	*Shaochong* HT 9, wood of the fire channel	*Dadun* LR 1, wood of the wood channel
	Excess	*Shenmen* HT 7, earth of the fire channel	*Taibai* SP 3, earth of the earth channel
Pericardium (fire)	Deficiency	*Zhongchong* PC 9, wood of the fire channel	*Dadun* LR 1, wood of the wood channel
	Excess	*Daling* PC 7, earth of the fire channel	*Taibai* SP 3, earth of the earth channel
Spleen (earth)	Deficiency	*Dadu* SP 2, fire of the earth channel	*Shaofu* HT 8, fire of the fire channel
	Excess	*Shangqiu* SP 5, metal of the earth channel	*Jingqu* LU 8, metal of the metal channel
Kidney (water)	Deficiency	*Fuliu* KI 7, metal of the water channel	*Jingqu* LU 8, metal of the metal channel
	Excess	*Yongquan* KI 1, wood of the water channel	*Dadun* LR 1, wood of the wood channel
Liver (wood)	Deficiency	*Ququan* LR 8, water of the wood channel	*Yingu* KI 10, water of the water channel
	Excess	*Xingjian* LR 2, fire of the wood channel	*Shaofu* HT 8, fire of the fire channel

The Lung (*Fei*)

The lung is associated with the metal phase. Its corresponding *fu* bowel is the large intestine, its tissue is the skin, its sense organ is the nose, its secretion is nasal mucus, and its outgrowth is the body hair. It is said to control the *qi*, exhalation, and the circulation of body fluids, especially in the upper body. It "descends and perfuses," and is said to "face the hundred vessels". In Biomedical terms, it comprises not only the ventilation function of the respiratory system, but also a part of the immune system, thermoregulation, and the opening and closing of the pores.

The lung is the *zang* located highest in the body (in the chest cavity, above the other organs), and is considered the most exterior of the *zang*. It absorbs the *qi* of air and transforms it into the *qi* that fuels bodily functions.

Lung Pathology Normal lung function permits the unobstructed circulation of *qi*, evidenced by even and harmonious breathing. A deficiency of lung *qi* manifests as feeble respiration, uneven breathing, weak speech, and lassitude. Normally, lung *qi*

Table 2.7 "Mother-Son" point combinations for deficiency and excess conditions of the *yang* channels

Channel	Condition	Affected channel ("Mother or Son Points")	"Mother-Son Channel" (element points)
Large intestine (metal)	Deficiency	*Quchi* LI 11, earth of the metal channel	*Zusanli* ST 36, earth of the earth channel
	Excess	*Erjian* LI 2, water of the metal channel	*Zutonggu* UB 66, water of the water channel
Small Intestine (fire)	Deficiency	*Houxi* SI 3, wood of the fire channel	*Zulinqi* GB 41, wood of the wood channel
	Excess	*Xiaohai* SI 8, earth of the fire channel	*Zusanli* ST 36, earth of the earth channel
Sanjiao (fire)	Deficiency	*Zhongzhu* SJ 3, wood of the fire channel	*Zulinqi* UB 41, wood of the wood channel
	Excess	*Tianjing* SJ 10, earth of the fire channel	*Zusanli* ST 36, earth of the earth channel
Stomach (earth)	Deficiency	*Jiexi* ST 41, fire of the earth channel	*Yanggu* SI 5, fire of the fire channel
	Excess	*Lidui* ST 45, metal of the earth channel	*Shangyang* LI 1, metal of the metal channel
Urinary bladder (water)	Deficiency	*Zhiyin* UB 67, metal of the water channel	*Shangyang* LI 1, metal of the metal channel
	Excess	*Shugu* UB 65, wood of the water channel	*Zulinqi* UB 41, wood of the wood channel
Gallbladder (wood)	Deficiency	*Xiaxi* UB 43, water of the wood channel	*Zutonggu* UB 66, water of the water channel
	Excess	*Yangfu* UB 38, fire of the wood channel	*Yanggu* SI 5, fire of the fire channel

descends. Loss of this function manifests as a replete sensation in the chest, cough, and shortness of breath. This may be caused by deficiency of lung *qi* or by obstruction caused by exterior pathogens attacking the body. The lung is also believed to maintain the body's defenses by ensuring circulation of *qi* close to the surface of the body. Loss of this function is evidenced by symptoms such as aversion to cold, fever, nasal obstruction, nasal discharge, cough, and wheezing or shortness of breath. In severe cases, it may manifest as asthma. It may also cause dry skin and hair. Deficiency of lung *qi* can also cause spontaneous sweating, while an obstruction of the lung's dispersing function will prevent sweating.

The Heart (*Xin*)

The heart is associated with the Fire phase. Its corresponding *fu* bowel is the small intestine, its tissue is the blood vessels, its sense organ is the tongue, its secretion is sweat, and its outgrowth is the facial complexion. It controls the circulation of blood and is the seat of mental activity. It is referred to as the "Emperor" or "ruler" of all the *zang*. In biomedical terms, the concept of *xin* encompasses the heart, the circulatory system and all blood vessels, and many functions of the higher nervous system.

Heart Pathology Deficiency of heart *qi* causes a feeble, weak pulse, or an irregular pulse, and a pale facial complexion. It can also cause stagnation of blood, which would then lend a bluish tint to the complexion and purplish coloration to the tongue. Deficiency of heart blood causes palpitations, insomnia, dream-disturbed sleep, poor memory, and restlessness, with a pale tongue. If a heat pathogen enters the blood, it will cause delirium, coma, anxiety, and similar symptoms, as well as a stiff tongue.

The Liver (*Gan*)

The liver is associated with the wood phase. Its corresponding *fu* bowel is the gallbladder, its tissue is the sinews (referring to the stiffer tissues of the joints and muscles, i.e., the continuum of periosteum, cartilage, tendon, fascial sheaths, and so on), its sense organ is the eyes, its secretion is tears, and its outgrowth is the nails. It is in charge of "coursing and discharging," "the unimpeded flow of *qi*," and "marshaling the blood," i.e., it manages the body's resources and the steady progression of all life processes. Because of this, the liver is also considered to be in charge of movement in the body and management of emotions. In biomedical terms, the TCM liver encompasses not only liver function but also emotional activities, volition, and autonomic muscle control.

Liver Pathology Disruption of the liver's command over blood can lead to hemorrhagic diseases, whereas deficiency of liver blood can manifest as vertigo, tremors or numbness of the extremities, or contracture or spasm of muscles and tendons, impairment of limb flexion and extension, scanty menstruation or absence of menstruation. Because the liver is in charge of managing the emotions as part of its coursing and discharging function, any affectation of the patient's emotional state is understood as a disruption of liver function. Liver *qi* stagnation, probably the most common pattern of disharmony in TCM practice, manifests with a plethora of symptoms, including fullness of the chest, feelings of frustration, discomfort in the hypochondrium, agitation, sadness, depression, irregular menstruation, and so on. Liver function may also become excessive, manifesting as irritability, insomnia, dream-disturbed sleep, dizziness, vertigo, ringing in the ears, or deafness. Any intense emotional upset, especially anger or mental depression, may impair the coursing and discharging function of the liver, leading to stagnation and any or all of the symptoms described above.

Liver function is intimately connected to the processes of digestion in TCM. Impairment of the free flow of *qi* readily affects the transportation and transformation functions of spleen and stomach (see below), causing jaundice, bitter taste in the mouth, distension and pain in the chest and hypochondrium, belching, and diarrhea.

Liver disharmony can also present with eye symptoms, including blurry vision, night blindness, or dryness. If a heat pathogen attacks the liver, redness, swelling, and pain of the eyes may result. Severe cases of this may also manifest with convulsions, opisthotonos, and lockjaw.

The Spleen (*Pi*)

The spleen is associated with the earth phase. Its associated *fu* bowel is the stomach, its tissue is the flesh (which refers to the cellular components of muscles, as opposed to the connective tissue membranes that make up the "sinews" that correspond to the liver), its sense organ is the mouth, its secretion is saliva, and its outgrowth is the lips. It is said to be in charge of "transportation and transformation," referring to the functions of digestion and assimilation of nutrients, as well as distribution of the products of digestion to all tissues of the body. The spleen is also charged with controlling the blood, keeping it within the blood vessels, and with ensuring that all organs remain in their place within the body cavity. In Western biomedicine, this encompasses the functions of the digestive system, particularly those of the small intestine, pancreas, and the liver that pertain to metabolizing and assimilating nutrients.

Spleen Pathology Failure of the spleen's function of transportation and transformation can manifest as abdominal distension, diarrhea, lassitude, emaciation, and malnutrition. Because this function controls the orderly movement of fluids inside the body, its deterioration can lead to the accumulation of pathological metabolites (known in TCM as *tan yin*) in the form of edema, watery diarrhea, or ascites. Easy bruising that takes a long time to heal, various types of internal bleeding, and frequent hemorrhages are signs of a breakdown of the spleen's function of controlling the blood. Malnutrition, muscular atrophy, and weakness of the limbs are symptoms of a deficiency of the spleen, as well as loss of appetite and marked fatigue after eating.

The Kidney (*Shen*)

The kidney is associated with the water phase. Its associated *fu* bowel is the bladder. Its tissue is the bones, its sense organ is the ear, its secretion is the urine, and its outgrowth is the hair of the head. It is considered the most *yin* of the *zang* because of its location in the inferior regions of the body and its command over the "essential substance" of the body, called *jing*, and which refers to the genetic inheritance received at conception. Furthermore, the kidney in TCM is the seat of the "Fire of the Gate of Vitality," that is, the original source of the motive force that propels all the body's functions. As such, it is said to be "the source of the original (*yuan*) *yin* and *yang*" of the body, in charge of providing the other organs with the resources to perform their proper functions. It is considered to be in charge of the functions of growth, development, and reproduction, as well as assisting the lungs in inhalation. In addition to the bones, the marrow and the brain are associated with the kidney.

In biomedical terms, the TCM kidney encompasses the metabolic functions of the kidney, those of the urogenital system, as well as genetic inheritance, endocrine function (particularly the thyroid and the pituitary–adrenal and pituitary–gonadal axes), and the ventilation function of the diaphragm.

Kidney Pathology As we have seen before (Sect. Yinyang theory), there is a very strong dependence and close interaction between the *yin* and *yang*, i.e., the structure and function, of the body. These are believed to have a common source in the kidney, and kidney pathology refers mainly to a deficiency in either the structural or functional aspects of the body. Infertility, deficient infantile development, malformations, congenital diseases, and poor bone structure all point to a deficiency of structure, i.e., kidney *yin*. Other manifestations of deficiency of *yin* that involve the kidney include soreness, aching, and weakness of the lumbar region and knees, blurred vision, and poor memory. If the deficiency of kidney *yin* causes an excess of metabolic activity, there will be tidal fever, night sweating, dizziness, ringing of the ears, seminal emissions at night, and excessive dreaming. Notice how many of these symptoms are also associated with deficiency of blood (see Sect. *The Liver*). This is because the blood pertains to *yin*. Thus, the close relationship of all organ systems in TCM, and the interdependence of *yinyang*, can be seen in the body.

Conversely, kidney *yang* deficiency relates to deterioration in function, and manifests as lassitude, coldness, and pain in the lumbar region and the knees, cold extremities, frequent urination and enuresis, or scanty urination and retention of urine. It is the cause of pathological conditions such as inadequate reproductive ability, impotence, premature ejaculation, and coldness of the uterus. Uneven breathing, dyspnea, and asthma are signs of the kidney losing its function of "grasping the *qi*," i.e., aiding respiration.

If either kidney *yin* or *yang* reaches a certain degree of depletion, it may injure the other and cause the physiological balance between structure and function in the body to be lost. Notice that in the absence of cold symptoms, kidney-related deterioration of function is sometimes called "kidney-*qi*" deficiency and symptoms of structural decay of the body associated with the kidney that do not also present heat symptoms are sometimes labeled as "kidney-essence" deficiency.

The Uterus The Uterus has a special status in TCM. It is considered an "extraordinary" *fu* organ, i.e., it is not associated with its own acupuncture channel, and although it is hollow like the rest of the *fu*, it stores blood temporarily and serves as the "palace of the fetus." Because of its role in reproduction, it is associated with the kidney. Symptoms of uterine dysfunction (irregular menstruation, absence of menstruation, and infertility) are often considered to be kidney (or liver) pathology.

The Six *Fu*

In contrast with the *zang*, which are solid in structure and in charge of various functions of storage and construction, the *fu* are said to be hollow, and their functions relate to the passage of substances through the body (mostly food). An adage in TCM goes, "The five *zang* store but do not drain; the six *fu* drain but do not store." Proper function of the *fu* implies constant motion. Their pathology is frequently keyed to obstruction of the free passage by various pathogens.

Briefly, the six *fu* and their functions are as follows:

- The stomach (*wei*), considered the "chief" of the *fu*, is in charge of receiving the food we eat. Its function is called the "rotting and ripening" of food and pertains to the initial stages of digestion. It is associated with the spleen.
- The small intestine (*xiao chang*) is understood as being in charge of separating "the clear from the turbid" along with the large intestine (*da chang*), which also oversees the formation and expulsion of stool. Although associated with the heart and the lung, respectively, their functions are more relevant to those of the spleen and stomach.
- The gallbladder (*dan*) stores bile and participates in the liver's coursing and discharging functions; in TCM, it is said to be associated with the capacity for resolve, decision-making, and taking action.
- The urinary bladder (*pang guang*) handles the expulsion of fluids managed by the kidney.
- The *sanjiao* is unique to TCM. Known as "the *fu* with function but no form," it is believed to be the "triple furnace" where the functions of the rest of the *zangfu* take place. The organs are housed within the three chambers of the *sanjiao* (upper, middle, and lower). The *sanjiao*, along with the lung, spleen, and kidney, is also in charge of "the waterways" of the body, i.e., its function involves the transmission of fluids throughout the body.

Theory of Channels and Collaterals (jingluo xue shuo)

TCM holds that *qi* and blood circulate throughout the body in a network of vessels known as channels and collaterals (*jingluo*). These serve as the connection between the interior and the exterior of the body, binding together all its parts into an integrated whole. The *jingluo* form a circuit, connecting the *zangfu* to each other and the extremities, the head, and the surface of the body. Twelve main channels (*jing*) exist that are associated with each of the *zangfu*. It is along their trajectories that acupuncture points are located. Each of these main channels has a myofascial tract (traditionally referred to as "sinew channel," *jing jin*), a deeper-lying "divergent" pathway (*jing bie*), and a collateral (*luo*) associated with it. In addition, deeper-lying vessels, known as the extraordinary vessels (*qi jing ba mai*), act as reservoirs for the twelve main channels, completing the system.

The twelve main channels receive a name according to their adscription to *yin* or *yang* (see Sect. Yinyang theory), their associated *zang* or *fu*, and the limb where their trajectory runs (arm or leg), as follows (presented in the order along which *qi* is said to proceed as it circulates through the body):

- Hand greater *yin* lung channel
- Hand *yang* brightness large intestine channel

- Foot *yang* brightness stomach channel
- Foot greater *yin* spleen channel
- Hand lesser *yin* heart channel
- Hand greater *yang* small intestine channel
- Foot greater *yang* bladder channel
- Foot lesser *yin* kidney channel
- Hand reverting *yin* pericardium channel
- Hand lesser *yang sanjiao* channel
- Foot lesser *yang* gallbladder channel
- Foot reverting *yin* liver channel

Among the eight extraordinary vessels, two deserve special mention because of their location along the midline of the body, along with the fact that they too have acupuncture points along their trajectory (the rest of the extraordinary vessels do not):

- The *ren* vessel
- The *du* vessel

Theory of Qi, Blood, Essence, and Body Fluids (qi xue jing jinye xue shuo)

Qi, blood (*xue*), essence (*jing*), and body fluids (*jinye*) are collectively known as the vital substances, because life depends on their activity and their existence and function are dependent on the vitality of the organism. All changes that occur in the body throughout life are the result of the interaction of the vital substances. *Zangfu* theory posits that circulation of *qi* and blood through the channels and networks connects the internal organs with the more superficial tissues and the body as a whole with its surroundings, constituting a unified whole. The activity of the *zangfu* simultaneously consumes and regenerates the body's stores of the vital substances.

The vital substances of TCM are a continuum, ranging from more to less substantial, underlying all of which is *qi* [12–15].

Qi

The concept of *qi* is one of the most pervasive in Chinese culture, yet translating the term into any other language is practically impossible. It has been explained as energy, material force, matter, ether, matter energy, life force, vital power, and moving power. *Qi* is fundamental and continuous and which exists as a result of the interaction between *yin* and *yang* since the beginning of the universe.

In TCM, *qi* is sometimes understood as a rarefied, metabolically active stuff that fills the vessels and propels blood and nourishes the body and fuels its vital activity. At others, it is the sum total of the system's activities, or the normal, physiological function of an organ or tissue.

Qi as the rarefied stuff in the channels and networks is said to be produced by the body's action on three sources: the essence (*jing*) received from the parents at conception and stored in the kidney, the "*qi* of grain and water" obtained by the spleen through the process of digestion, and the *qi* derived from the air breathed in through the lung.

The functions of this *qi* are as follows:

- To promote activity, growth, and development, fueling the activity of the *zangfu* and other tissues, propel the circulation of blood through the vessels and distribute fluids to all tissues.
- To warm the body and maintain normal body temperature.
- To protect the surface of the body against pathogens (*xie qi*). In this capacity, *qi* is known as upright *qi* (*zheng qi*), sometimes also referred to as "anti-pathogenic" *qi*.
- Stabilize and bind, ensure stability of the tissues and the proper position of all body structures, contain the blood within the vessels, and regulate loss of fluids, such as urine, sweat, saliva, and semen.
- Mobilize and transform. The constant motion of *qi* is described as "ascending, descending, exiting, and entering." Normal physiology assumes harmonious movement in all directions. Its action ensures the production and correct consumption of blood, essence, and body fluids.

Original *Qi* (*Yuan Qi*) Original *qi* arises from the prenatal essence received at conception. It constitutes the original impetus of life and promotes normal activity in all organs and tissues. It is said to be the basis of resistance to disease and the extension of life into longevity. Its pathology relates mainly to chronic, debilitating disease, weakened *zangfu* function, premature aging, and reduced resistance to disease. It is circulated mainly through the *sanjiao* and the extraordinary vessels.

Chest *Qi* (*Zong Qi*) Chest *qi* is the result of the interaction between the *qi* acquired through respiration and the "*qi* of water and grain" obtained through digestion. It arises in the thorax, penetrates the heart vessels, and descends to pour into the lower limbs. Its main function is regulation of the activity of the lung and heart, and is responsible for appropriate circulation of *qi* and blood throughout the body. Chest *qi* also connects with the extraordinary vessel known as the thoroughfare (*chong*) to aid in providing the uterus with adequate blood supply to promote menstruation. Chest *qi* pathology relates mainly to lung disease, especially *qi* deficiency, as well as cardiovascular diseases, diseases of the peripheral circulation, pain in the chest, menstrual irregularities, and pain and weakness of the legs.

Nutritive *Qi* (*Ying Qi*) Nutritive *qi* is the result of the transformation of food. It circulates through the twelve regular channels and then enters the *du* and *ren* extraordinary vessels at the throat. It is the main kind of *qi* involved in transformation and production of blood. It is a constituent of blood and provides nourishment to the body. Its pathology relates mostly to diseases of the spleen and stomach, especially blood deficiency, spleen *qi* deficiency, and obstruction of *qi* and blood in the channels.

Defensive *Qi* (*Wei Qi*) Also obtained from the "*qi* of water and grain," defensive *qi* circulates outside the vessels. It is in charge of protection of the body at the surface, opening and closing of the pores, regulating body temperature, warming the body, and moistening the skin. Its action is said to relate to circadian rhythms and cycles of sleeping and waking. Its pathology pertains mostly to diseases caused by external pathogens, recurrent upper respiratory tract diseases, disorders of the skin, sweating, regulation of body temperature, and sleep disturbances.

Pathology of *Qi*

- *Qi* deficiency: respiratory diseases and decreased body resistance (lung), diseases of blood, digestive tract, and genitals (spleen), decreased immunity, and chronic and degenerative diseases (kidney)
- *Qi* sinking: prolapsed and chronic diarrhea (spleen)
- *Qi* stagnation: hepatobiliary, gastrointestinal, and genitourinary diseases, pain, tumors, emotional disorders (liver and spleen)
- *Qi* counterflow: nausea, vomiting, hiccup, belching, heartburn, acid reflux, cough, asthma, headache, vertigo, and so on (lung, liver, and stomach)

Blood (*Xue*)

Blood arises as a result of the transformation of food by the spleen, assisted by kidney essence. It flows constantly in the vessels, propelled by *qi*, and under the direction of the liver and the command of the heart. Its main functions are to nourish and lubricate, making sinew and bones strong and keeping the joints flexible. Blood is said to be the "Residence of the Mind," i.e., the foundation for mental and emotional activity in the body.

Blood pathology pertains mainly to the spleen, liver, and heart, and is of one of three types: deficiency, stagnation, or heat. It may manifest as menstrual irregularities, painful menstruation, uterine fibroids, endometriosis, fixed, stabbing pains anywhere in the body, tumors, circulatory disorders, hemorrhagic diseases, poor memory, emotional disorders, dry and brittle nails, hair, skin, constipation, fatigue.

Essence (*Jing*)

Essence in TCM is a refined substance, initially received by the fetus at conception from the parents and then stored by the kidney and used as a resource for growth, development, and reproduction throughout life. This is called "prenatal" essence and is deemed to be a finite, irreplaceable resource. The functional activity of the *zangfu*, especially the spleen and stomach, creates and replenishes a secondary store of essence known as "postnatal" essence, which maintains life and fuels its processes. Kidney essence strengthens the bones, produces the bone marrow, and nourishes the brain. Essence pathology relates to hereditary diseases, developmental disorders, and degenerative diseases, diseases of the brain, cerebrovascular system, reproductive organs, and bones, and disorders of the sense organs (especially the ears). Overindulgence in sexual activity is seen as damaging to the essence and can be the cause of deterioration in other systems as well.

Body Fluids (*Jinye*)

The term *jinye* refers collectively to all the fluids of the body other than blood and semen (which is considered part of *jing*, see Sect. Essence). It includes secretions, such as saliva, gastrointestinal juices, synovial fluid, tears, mucus, sweat, and urine.

Jin is the clearer, lighter, thinner, and less dense portion of bodily fluids. *Jin* fluids are *yang*, as compared with *ye* fluids (sometimes translated as "humors") which are *yin*, i.e., more turbid, heavier, and denser. *Jin* fluids are relatively more watery and fluid and have functions relating to lubrication of skin and muscles and strengthening and nourishing of skin, akin to the defensive *qi* (Sect. Defensive *qi* (*wei qi*)). *Ye* humor, on the other hand, is said to be poured into the joints, brain, spinal cord, and sensory organs, which it lubricates and strengthens, in a way akin to the functions of nutritive *qi*.

Formation, distribution, and excretion of body fluids proceed from the digestion of food in the stomach and intestines. The essential fluids are absorbed and transported by the spleen to the chest, whereas the turbid waste is excreted with the feces. Essential fluid is then distributed by the action of the heart and lung to the organs and tissues of the body. The kidney excretes surplus fluid as urine, while the opening and closing of the pores allows fluids to escape the body in the form of sweat.

Body fluids accumulate because of diminished function of the organs in charge of fluid metabolism, i.e., lung, spleen, and kidney. Pathology of the body fluids includes deficiency caused by excessive consumption (by heat pathogens) or loss (sweating, diarrhea, polyuria, vomiting, or bleeding), and abnormalities in circulation, which give rise to phlegm-rheum (*tan yin*), stagnation, damp-turbidity, fluid retention, edema, and so on.

Etiology and Pathophysiology in Traditional Chinese Medicine

As has been emphasized, TCM has a unique way of looking at health and illness. It does not rely on animistic or magical explanations for disease causation, yet it also does not recognize the existence of pathogens the way Western biomedicine does. From a TCM perspective, the virus or bacterium is not the causative agent per se, but one of the intermediate contributing factors for development of disease. According to TCM theory, the fundamental factor in etiology is weakness of the body's normal function, referred to as *zheng qi*. Once *zheng qi* has been weakened for whatever reason (sudden weather changes, emotional upsets, overexertion, poor eating habits, and so on), particular conditions arise that manifest as dysfunction. Disease thus arises when the balance of the body's processes (structure and function, *qi* and blood, *zangfu*, and the channel system) is lost. In lieu of this initial disharmony, says TCM theory, no disease can arise. The *Neijing Suwen*, the oldest extant text on TCM theory, says "*Yin* is calm, *yang* is hidden, therefore the spirit is at rest." This condition of balance extends to the relationship between the body and its surrounding environment. Quoting from the *Suwen* again, "*Yinyang* of the four seasons are the beginning and end of all things, the root of life and death. To go against them damages life; to follow their course prevents the arisal of disease." TCM thus classifies pathogenic factors according to their origin:

Exogenous Also known as "the six weather evils" (*liu yin*), these are wind (*feng*), cold (*han*), damp (*shi*), dryness (*zao*), summer heat (*shu*), and heat (*re*). Also classified in this category is pestilential *qi* (*li qi*), i.e., epidemic diseases.

Endogenous The "seven emotions" (*qi qing*) (anger, euphoria, worry, sadness, fear, melancholy, and fright) are said to adversely affect the flow of *qi*, thus giving rise to disharmony and disease.

Miscellaneous "Neither exogenous nor endogenous," this category includes all aspects of a disorderly lifestyle, such as poor diet, binging and starving, fatigue due to physical or mental overexertion, and excessive sexual activity. It also includes traumatic injury, parasites, poisonous bites, poisoning, and incorrect medical treatment. There are also the so-called "secondary pathogenic factors, such as blood stasis (*xue yu*) and phlegm (*tan*), which arise as the result of the others, but which in turn cause or complicate disease conditions.

Exogenous Pathogens: The Six Evils (Liu Yin/Liu Xie)

The exogenous pathogens are those that attack the body from the exterior and include the so called "six weather evils" and "pestilential *qi*." The ancient Chinese sages observed the effects of exposure on the human body, and determined that six climactic conditions could affect the *yinyang* balance of the organism. These six influences, namely wind, cold, damp, dryness, summer heat, and heat, adversely affect health when they change suddenly and surpass the body's capacity to adapt or when preexisting imbalance makes the body susceptible to their pathogenic effects. Put otherwise, these influences are part of nature. It is only when they occur abruptly or when the organism is already weakened that they become etiological factors.

Under certain circumstances, pathological changes can induce conditions that resemble the symptoms caused by the external pathogenic influences. In such cases, one speaks of "internal dampness," "internal cold," "internal heat," "internal wind," and so on.

Wind (*Feng*)

Wind is characterized by a sudden onset and quick subsidence, lesions that shift location, and/or aversion to drafts. When affecting the skin, wind diseases cause itching. Other wind disease symptoms may include involuntary movement (twitching, tremors, and convulsions) or the sensation of abnormal movement (vertigo and dizziness).

Cold (*Han*)

Cold diseases are characterized by sensations of chills and or cold, muscular contraction, and localized pain that worsens with exposure to cold.

Dampness (*Shi*)

Dampness is associated with lingering illness, heaviness of body and limbs, or headache that feels as if the head is tightly bound. There may be turbidity in body excretions, such as leucorrhea, turbid urine, and exudates from skin lesions. There can be sensations of fullness or distension in the abdomen, loss of appetite, nausea, vomiting, and loose stools, and in some cases, accumulation of fluids in the body, as in edema.

Dryness (*Zao*)

Dryness manifests as dry mouth, dry nose, dry throat, and dry cough.

Heat (*Re*)

Heat manifests as fever, thirst, scanty concentrated urine, constipation, a red tongue with yellow or no coating, and a rapid pulse. There may also be low fever in the afternoon, sensation of heat in the palms and soles, malar flush, and night sweating.

Fire (*Huo*)

Fire represents a stronger degree of heat and can manifest as acute inflammation and localized redness, swelling, sensation of heat, and pain, fever, restlessness, thirst, foul breath, bitterness in the mouth, ulceration of the tongue, and constipation, bleeding (epistaxis, hematuria, and so on), and/or a dark red tongue with a yellow, prickly coating, and rapid replete pulse. Diseases caused by endogenous fire are similar to those caused by endogenous heat, but may be accompanied by irritability and insomnia.

Endogenous Pathogens: The Seven Emotions (qi qing)

TCM treats excessive or unbalanced emotions as disease-causing factors because, through the systemic correspondences of five-phase theory, they are directly related to the *zangfu* organ systems. Each of the five *zang* is keyed to one emotion (see Table 2.2). The emotions are held to directly affect the movement of *qi* in specific ways which, like the six evils, may become pathogenic under given circumstances.

Emotions are a natural part of human existence, and no human being is above experiencing them. Under normal circumstances, emotions occur in response to outside stimuli, produce an effect, and pass quickly. Emotions become the cause of disease only when they are intense, violent, or continue for long periods. This is sometimes termed "over-excitement of the emotions" in that the emotions exceed the adaptive, regulatory capability of the body. They can impair *zangfu* function, perturb the *qi* dynamic, and upset the *yinyang* balance, thus leading to the development of pathological conditions.

Because they are generated from within, emotions readily injure the *zangfu*. As previously mentioned, each of the emotions is keyed to one of the *zang*, which it said to injure directly when in excess: euphoria injures the heart, anger injures the liver, sadness injures the lung, worry injures the spleen, and fear and fright injure the kidney. In addition, those organ systems directly in charge of mental/emotional activity, i.e., the heart and the liver, are affected by all pathological affects. The liver is directly in charge of coursing and discharging the emotions; a deterioration of this function causes the emotions to become more extreme. On the other hand, because the heart is the seat of mental activities, impairment or obstruction of this function will cause mania and depression.

As previously mentioned, the emotions perturb the movement of *qi*. Each of the emotions causes *qi* to move in a particular way, disturbing the *qi* dynamic on which the body depends to maintain harmony and balance. The disturbances of *qi* flow brought on by the emotions are summarized in Table 2.8, and explained later.

Anger induces *qi* to flow upward: the liver is the *zang* most readily affected by anger. When this happens, liver *qi* flows upward in excess, causing blood to move pathologically in this direction as well. This will manifest as a red face and eyes, dizziness and vertigo, distending pain of the head, or even sudden coma or syncope. Sometimes, hematemesis and diarrhea may also be observed as a result of blood following the adverse upward *qi* flow or a counterflow that attacks the spleen.

Euphoria relaxes the flow of *qi*: euphoria is excessive joy. Under normal circumstances, joy is desirable in that it promotes the harmonious flow of *qi* and blood. However, taken to excess, it causes poor concentration and mania.

Sadness consumes *qi*: Affecting the lung and its command of breathing, sadness as a pathogenic factor manifests as chest oppression and a demoralized attitude. Crying and weeping exhaust the *qi* and cause lassitude.

Worry causes *qi* to accumulate: Discursive thought requires *qi* to become fixed. When it becomes lengthy or intense, thinking easily becomes worry and causes *qi* to stagnate. Worry most readily injures the spleen, and thus, the manifestations of injury by worry include poor appetite, abdominal distension, constipation, and/or diarrhea.

Table 2.8 Effect of the emotions on the movement of *qi*

Emotion	Effect
Anger	*Qi* ascends
Euphoria	*Qi* relaxes
Worry	*Qi* accumulates
Sadness	*Qi* consumes
Fear	*Qi* descends
Fright	*Qi* disperses and moves recklessly

Fear causes *qi* to flow downward: Because the kidney is the *zang* in charge of urination and defecation, when fear injures it, there will be incontinence. Other manifestations include pain and weakness in the legs and knees as the function of the kidney to nourish the bones is impaired.

Fright causes *qi* to disperse: Sudden fear has the effect of causing the *qi* to collapse. This is seen as palpitations, anxiety or distress, and an inability to concentrate.

Because emotional overexcitation causes a breakdown of the normal flow of *qi*, it will invariably cause stagnation. Over time, any obstruction or accumulation of *qi* leads to internal heat and fire. This is commonly seen in the clinic. Patients with long-term emotional problems usually display some of the symptoms associated with the fire pathogen (see previous section). Key diagnostic signs are a red or crimson, dry tongue, possibly with a swollen and red tip, and a rapid and/or slippery pulse.

By the same token, emotions may also worsen a preexisting disease through their alteration of the *qi* dynamic. For example, a patient with hypertension (a disease caused by excessive rising of liver *yang* due to deficiency of both kidney and liver *yin*) may suffer from sudden coma or syncope, or even paralysis, after an incident of sudden and violent rage. This is because the liver is readily affected by anger, and sudden anger will induce rising of liver *yang*.

Conversely, as body, mind, and emotions are an integral and indivisible unit, it is equally likely for the process to occur in reverse, i.e., instead of the emotions causing disease, an organic disturbance may cause alteration of the emotions. For example, a state of protracted fear and anxiety will damage and weaken the kidney. On the other hand, if there is a deficiency of the kidney, due to having had multiple pregnancies and childbirths, the condition may also manifest with abnormal states of fear and anxiety. Frequently, a vicious cycle is established, where the emotion will feed the organic imbalance, which, in turn, favors the imbalanced emotional state that worsens or aggravates it, such as when a liver imbalance makes a person irritable, which in turn aggravates the liver imbalance.

In summary, when thinking of the emotions as pathogenic influences, they are said to damage the interior and perturb the flow of *qi* of the *zangfu*. They arise and are keyed to the *zangfu* and, under normal circumstances, will cause no damage as they are depurated by the liver's coursing and discharging. However, in excess, each of the emotions can affect one or more of the *zangfu*, causing pathological changes. Conversely, pathological changes in one of the *zangfu* may make one more prone to the emotion keyed to the affected organ system, which can create a vicious cycle of reinforcing disease-causing conditions.

Emotions in TCM and Psychosomatic Disease in Biomedicine

Western biomedicine concerns itself with organic alterations that are keyed to the physical structures of the interior of the body. When confronted with emotional symptoms, biomedicine deems them as beyond its scope of diagnosis and treatment. When symptoms are keyed to the patient's emotional state and no clear organic alterations can be found, biomedicine labels these cases as "psychosomatic" and refers them for psychiatric care. The unfortunate reality is that biomedicine conceives the emotions as being separate from the body and dismisses emotional manifestations as ultimately irrelevant to the origin, development, and outcome of a disease process.

TCM, however, views the emotions as an integral part of what constitutes health. Alterations of organ system function include the emotions, and a person is not understood to be healthy if their emotions are in an abnormal, imbalanced, or excessive state. For example, if there is an imbalance of the spleen and stomach, symptoms such as diarrhea or constipation, vomiting, nausea, poor appetite, heartburn, bloating, and abdominal pain will ensue, but these will likely be accompanied by states of anguish, anxiety, worry, lassitude, heaviness of the head and difficulty concentrating. Treatment would be aimed at correcting the spleen–stomach imbalance as a whole, and the emotional states would be seen to disappear along with the organic manifestations.

It is thereby clear how TCM theory embraces a holistic perspective. The body is made up of a group of interrelated systems that stand in functional relationship to each other in order to maintain balance and harmony. Each of these systems partakes of all dimensions of human experience (corporal, emotional, mental) simultaneously, as part of a continuum. Alteration of function can have multiple manifestations, some at the emotional level, others at the physical, but they all pertain to the same organ systems. The correlation of symptoms and signs occurring simultaneously is what allows for accurate diagnosis and, consequently, effective treatment.

Miscellaneous Pathogenic Factors (Nonexternal/Noninternal)

In addition to exogenous and endogenous pathogens, TCM recognizes other mechanisms whereby disease may develop, mostly related to lifestyle. This category also includes parasites, poisonous bites and substances, iatrogenic disease, and the so-called "secondary pathogenic influences," which are intermediate by-products of dysfunction that, in turn, can cause characteristic disease states.

Lifestyle Factors

Proper diet, work, appropriate regular exercise, and rest are imperative for human life and preservation of health. Improper diet as well as imbalances in activity (including sexual activity) will disturb the physiological functions of the body, leading to disease.

Improper Diet Improper dietary habits include undereating and overeating, eating excessive amounts of "cold" and/or "hot" foods, and disorderly eating. Insufficient eating will lead to deficiencies of *qi* and blood. Additionally, the body's *zheng qi* will be weakened from the lack of substance, making the body susceptible to invasion by exterior pathogens.

Overeating, in contrast, weakens the spleen and stomach, causing abdominal distension, epigastric pain, nausea, vomiting, burping, gastric reflux, and diarrhea. It may also induce food stagnation (indigestion) and, over time, malnutrition. It may also induce stagnation of blood and *qi* in the networks of the stomach and intestines, which manifests as bloody stools and/or bleeding hemorrhoids. Like all forms of stagnation, food stagnation that persists over time will transform into heat and subsequently into phlegm (see below).

Excessive consumption of sweet foods obstructs the transportation and transformation functions of the spleen, engendering internal dampness, which manifests as copious nasal discharge, abdominal distension and pain, mucus in the stool, and vaginal discharge. Excessive consumption of greasy, fatty foods such as deep-fried foods, dairy, bananas, peanuts, and fatty meats can also induce the formation of phlegm and dampness. These internal pathogens obstruct the spleen and cause sinusitis, nasal discharge, a sensation of heaviness in the body, dull pains, and a sensation of "fogginess" in the head.

TCM classifies foods (and medicinal substances) in terms of their "hot" or "cold" energetic quality. Raw vegetables and foods that are actually cold to the touch can injure the spleen and stomach, causing symptoms such as diarrhea, chills, cold phlegm, and abdominal distension and pain. On the other hand, rich, spicy, high-glycemic-index foods, and alcohol are considered hot and can cause stagnation and the appearance of internally generated heat in various points in the digestive tract.

Finally, eating in a hurry, arguing while eating, returning to work immediately after eating, late-night snacking, and eating while emotionally upset are all circumstances that injure the *yin* aspect of the stomach, manifesting as thirst, epigastric pain, and dry stools with a red tongue without coating in the center.

Imbalances Between Work and Rest Appropriate physical activity promotes the flow of *qi* and blood in the channels and strengthens the constitution. Proper rest relieves fatigue and restores mental and physical strength. However, excesses in either of these will disrupt the balance of the body and lead to disease.

Overexertion is activity; therefore, it pertains to *yang*. In excess, it injures the *qi* of kidney and spleen. Excessive mental work (akin to the worry emotion) readily damages the spleen, whereas excessive physical activity can damage the heart.

Conversely, excessive inactivity damages the flow of *qi* and blood and, over time, causes damage to the spleen and stomach, leading to generalized *qi* deficiency and the presence of dampness and phlegm, as in obesity.

Excessive Sexual Activity: A subjective condition to define, what constitutes "excessive" sexual activity is entirely dependent on the person's lifestyle, age, and current situation. Young, healthy individuals can certainly engage in sexual activity more often and intensely than old, frail ones. Regardless, TCM theory recognize signs that may be attributed to excessive sexual activity: fatigue, dizziness, blurred vision, painful and weak knees and lower back, frequent urination, reduced appetite, and reduced libido or erectile dysfunction in men. Sexual taxation damages primarily the kidney, as it is the *zang* associated with reproduction. This may manifest as seminal emission, impotence in men and menstrual irregularities in women, vaginal discharge, infertility, and frigidity. Also, because the kidney is the basis of the *jing*-essence acquired from the parents at conception, excessive sexual activity may induce premature aging or debility. Furthermore, sexual activity while exhausted or emotionally perturbed, or while intoxicated, will also damage the essence.

Traumatic Injury

According to TCM, traumatic injury causes localized stagnation of *qi* and blood. Even after a lesion has healed, localized weakening of the tissues surrounding the site of injury often remains, and pain and weakness of the area may occur again when old age, cold exposure, malnutrition, or further lesions weaken the flow of *qi* and blood in the area again. The category of trauma includes animal bites and burns.

Parasites

"Parasites" in TCM is an older disease category. It refers mostly to the presence of visible parasites, such as roundworm, ringworm, tapeworm, and the like.

Iatrogenic Diseases

Inadequate doses or wrongfully indicated pharmaceutical drugs can cause disease. Even when correctly indicated, pharmaceutical drugs can and frequently do have secondary side effects, which are covered under this category. Wrong diagnosis in the practice of TCM herbal medicine can also cause iatrogenic symptoms, although to a lesser degree and are easily corrected.

Secondary Pathogens

Disease in the body may lead to the appearance of pathological substances, which in turn become the cause of other symptoms. These are termed secondary or intermediate pathogens, and include *qi* stagnation (*qi zhi*), blood stasis (*xue yu*), and phlegm (*tan*).

- *Qi* stagnation is the cause of a variety of conditions marked by pain. A TCM adage states that "Wherever there is obstruction, there will be pain." Pain attributed to *qi* stagnation is accompanied by distension and has no clear, fixed location. *Qi* stagnation may also be specific to one or more of the *zangfu*, perturbing their function directly.
- Blood stasis is considered the cause of a large number of pathological changes, chief of which is extravasation as the flow becomes impeded and blood escapes the vessels. Congestion, thrombosis, ischemia, hepatomegaly, splenomegaly, and many types of tumors are attributed to blood stasis as well. Blood stasis is also associated with pain; however, this pain is severe, stabbing, and sharp. The patient can easily pinpoint its location. Blood stasis conditions are evidenced by purplish colorations in the tongue and elsewhere in the body.
- Phlegm is a concept that deserves particular attention in TCM. The result of long-term stagnation and ensuing internal heat, a loss of the transformation function of the spleen and/or a breakdown of the kidney's command of the turbid fluids of the body, phlegm in TCM encompasses more than just the turbid discharge of the nasal passages. It is the cause of "the hundred strange diseases," and may manifest as vomiting, cough with dyspnea and expectoration, numbness, facial paralysis, enlargement of the lymph nodes, palpitations, shortness of breath, and even manic behavior and loss of consciousness.

References

1. Temelie B. The five-elements wellness plan. A Chinese system for perfect health. New York: Sterling; 2002.
2. Junying G, Zhihong S. Practical traditional Chinese medicine and pharmacology, basic theories and principles. Beijing: New World Press; 1990.
3. Yubin L, Chengcai L. Advanced TCM Series. Concepts and theories of traditional Chinese medicine. Vol. 2. Beijing: Science Press; 1997.
4. Zhu-Fan X. Best of traditional Chinese medicine. Beijing: New World Press; 1995.
5. Marié E. Compendio de Medicina China. Fundamentos, Teoría y Práctica. Original title, Précis de Médicine Chinoise. S.A. Madrid, Spain: EDAF; 1998.
6. Jianping H. Methodology of traditional Chinese medicine. Beijing: New World Press; 1995.
7. Compiled by Beijing College of Traditional Chinese Medicine. Shanghai College of Traditional Chinese Medicine. Nanjing College of Traditional Chinese Medicine. The Acupuncture Institute of the Academy of Traditional Chinese Medicine. Essentials of Chinese acupuncture. Beijing, China: Foreign Languages Press; 1980.
8. Ross J, Zang F. The organ systems of traditional Chinese medicine. Philadelphia: 2nd ed. Elsevier Churchill Livingstone; 1985.

9. Kaptchuk TJ. The web that has no weaver. New York: McGraw-Hill; 2000.
10. Porkert M. The theoretical foundations of Chinese medicine. System of correspondence. Cambridge: The MIT Press; 1978.
11. Maciocia G. The foundations of Chinese medicine. Philadelphia: 2nd ed. Elsevier Churchill Livingstone; 2005.
12. Xuesheng Z. Zhongyi jiqu lilun tubiaojie Chinese "Medicine Basic Theory Chart Explanations". Renmin weisheng chubanshe. Beijing: People's Medical Publishing House; 2004.
13. Yimin L. Zhongyi Jichu Lilun Shiyao "Chinese Medicine Basic Theory Essential Explanations". Zhongyi guji chubanshe. Beijing: Chinese Medicine Ancient Books Press; 1997.
14. Xiaohui H. Zhongyi Jichu lilun. Traditional Chinese medicine basic theory No. 2 Renmin weisheng chubanshe. Beijing: People's Medical Publishing House; 2010.
15. Xing J. Zhongyi Jichu Lilun Yixue Zhukao Koudai Congshu. Chinese Medicine Foundations easy study test pocket book series. Zhongguo Zhongyiyao Chubanshe. Beijing: China's Chinese Medicine Press; 2004.

Chapter 3
Pattern Discrimination in Traditional Chinese Medicine (TCM)

Francisco Lozano

Introduction

Pattern discrimination is a unique diagnostic system used in the practice of traditional Chinese medicine (TCM). It is intended to provide clear identification of the condition of a patient in an individualized manner. It can be applied to the diagnosis of a specific disease or clearly defined pathological condition. However, it can also be used to define the overall health condition of a relatively healthy person without any major complaints, including tendencies that may lead to disease if left unaddressed.

Traditional Chinese Medicine offers a unique approach to diagnosis and categorization of illnesses, called "pattern discrimination."

In order to better understand the importance and usefulness of pattern discrimination in the practice of acupuncture and TCM, it is necessary to review the concept of diagnosing disease, as well as comparing and contrasting the views of both TCM and Western biomedical paradigms regarding diagnosis. We shall also look at theories and concepts that support the process of diagnosis and treatment.

Diagnosis in Western Biomedicine

The Universal Concept of Medical Diagnosis

> Diagnosis is the identification of the nature and cause of anything, the art or act of identifying a disease from its signs and symptoms

F. Lozano (✉)
Medical Acupuncture Specialty, National School of Medicine & Homeopathy, National Polytechnic Institute, Guillermo Massieu Helguera Num. 239, Fraccionamiento la Escalera, Ticomán, Mexico D.F., Mexico
e-mail: lozanof57@gmail.com

In the practice of any form of medicine, diagnosis is one of the most important steps to accomplishing the correct treatment to cure, alleviate suffering, or prevent disease from developing. Without precise diagnosis, it is almost impossible to proceed with an appropriate treatment strategy.

No Diagnosis = No Treatment

In the absence of a clear diagnosis, the medical practitioner cannot effect a treatment that will clearly address the patient's condition. At best, the physician will provide symptomatic or palliative treatment to relieve suffering partially and/or temporarily. In Western biomedicine, correct diagnosis primarily relies on attaining confirmation of the cause and recognition of the main pathological process, which is usually established and expected from previous experience. Absence of a complete set of evidence with confirmation from laboratory, imaging, and other specialized tests precludes establishing a definitive diagnosis. This makes choosing a corresponding treatment modality difficult.

Diagnosis as Necessary Label, Diagnosis as "Box"

Western biomedical diagnosis frequently relies upon "labeling" diseases. Patients who fit certain parameters of a disease are labeled as having that disease, and will receive the standard treatment given for that disease, with little or no adjustment to fit individual conditions. Practitioners of biomedicine are then confronted with the clinical reality that each patient responds differently to conventional treatment. This frequently leads to reconsideration of the original diagnosis, "imprecise" diagnoses, or the use of nonspecific, symptomatic treatments aimed at ameliorating the problem at hand [1].

Foundations of TCM Diagnosis

To understand TCM pattern discrimination, it is crucial to review some basic concepts and theoretical underpinnings of Chinese medical theory. TCM theory is characterized by a peculiar approach to diagnosis and treatment that applies a series of flexible, individualized parameters based on a naturalistic, integrative view. TCM does not use complicated or aggressive procedures to confirm a diagnosis, instead relying mainly on the careful analysis and interpretation of information obtained through various forms of patient observation.

One of the basic theoretical pillars that supports the TCM system is the concept of the "body as an integrated unity" (*zheng ti guan nian*) or "whole body system." According to this view, all external expressions of the condition of the body are observed and compared with the external environment and then analyzed systematically to explain what is occurring inside the body of the patient [2–6].

TCM Diagnosis and the "Black Box" Model

The TCM diagnostic model could well be likened to the so-called Black Box model, which seeks to determine the contents of the black box without opening it, through the application of external stimuli and appreciation of external reactions. Following this analogy, the body is the black box and what is going on inside is determined (i.e., diagnosed) through what comes out of the box (signs and symptoms, pulse and tongue images, facial complexion, feces, etc.). The salient feature of this model is that it preserves the integrity of the whole system.

This concept is expressed in the chapter "The Foundation of the Organs" (*Lingshu ben zang*) in the Neijing, one of the oldest sources of Chinese medical theory, specifically in the following expressions: "All what is in the inside, reflects on the outside" and "The inspection of the exterior lets you determine the state of the internal organs, then you can know what kind of disease affects the patient."

The Holistic or Integral Concept of TCM (Zheng Ti Guan Nian)

The concept of holism in TCM has two aspects: the body as an integrated whole and the unity of man and nature. TCM views the human body as an organic whole. Although the body is composed of various tissues, all parts and functions of the body—organs, channels, vital substances, etc.—are always connected to each other, functioning as a unity. Furthermore, the human being is an active part of the whole universe. On one hand, the natural world constantly influences the body, and on the other, the body adapts to conform to variations in the natural environment [7–9].

No part of the whole is isolated, all are mutually related. Therefore, when there is a disturbance in one region, sooner or later it will affect other parts of the whole. According to TCM, the disruptions caused to the adaptation process of the organism by those disturbances are the origin of disease.

The Five Phases and the Organic-Energetic Systems

The five-phase system is another theoretical construct of classical Chinese naturalistic thought that reflects the holistic concept when applied to TCM. This system establishes functional correspondences between various natural phenomena under the main categories of the five phases. These are water, wood, fire, metal, and water. Five phase theory applied to TCM recognizes five main "depots" (*zang*), the most

Table 3.1 Organic-energetic systems (five levels)

Five levels	Five-element system				
	1. Water	2. Wood	3. Fire	4. Earth	5. Metal
1. Body structure	Bones	Sinews	Vessels	Muscles	Skin
2. Organ	Kidney	Liver	Heart	Spleen	Lung
3. Sense organ	Ears	Eyes	Tongue	Mouth	Body hair
4. Emotion	Fear	Anger	Joy	Thoughtfulness	Melancholy
5. Spiritual mental activity	Will	Courage	Ideation	Consciousness	Instinct

important organs in the body (namely, lung, liver, heart, spleen, and kidneys), and the rest of the tissues of the body (structures, internal organs, sense orifices, emotions, and spiritual/mental functions) are organized into systems under the aegis of these *zang* organs, each of which is linked to one of these five phases by virtue of their functional relationships (see Table 3.1). This system of relationships extends to pathology and treatment. When one component of one of the organ systems is diseased, the disease is said to "pertain" or be the province of the corresponding organ. Acupuncture points are in turn associated with each of the *zang* organs and can be chosen to treat disorders affecting their associated tissues/body structures. For example, a disease affecting the bones could be treated using acupuncture points on the kidney channel. Moreover, diseases in one part of these organ systems are frequently seen to affect its other parts. In our example, the patient may also report discomfort in the ears and lack of willpower to act.

Holistic Approach of TCM Diagnosis and Practice

TCM stresses the need for a holistic approach to treating illness. Patients are not divided into parts, where every condition is localized and diagnosed separately, with a specialist required to deal with each part and individual condition and treatments that may frequently be at odds with each other. Chinese medical thought calls for a therapeutic strategy that keeps sight of the patient's overall health, addressing all symptoms and complaints as part of one disease process. This produces faster, superior, and more appreciable effects for patients.

Individualized Diagnosis

Individualized diagnosis and treatment constitute an important principle of TCM. In the practice of Chinese medicine, diagnosis and treatment are always performed with the patients' age, gender, constitution, and lifestyle in mind, as well as the presentation and evolution of the disease (pattern discrimination).

Dynamic Balance Between Health and Disease

Classical Chinese thought holds that all phenomena in the universe are moving and changing continuously. This is true in TCM, where the physiological phenomena of the human body are perceived to be a process of constant transformation and interaction. Normal physiological and pathological conditions are a pattern of continuous flux. It is this dynamic balance that maintains health, and disease is seen as a deviation from the correct evolution of this pattern.

Diagnosis Adjusts to the Dynamic Process of Disease

It follows, then, that disease is not a static picture in this system. TCM regards disease as a dynamic process, continuously changing and adjusting to environmental, dietary, emotional, and other factors attendant to the situation of the patient. Thus, diagnosis and treatment need to be continuously adjusted to the evolution of the disease dynamic for each individual patient.

TCM Diagnosis

The Four Methods/The Patient File/Relevant Information According to TCM

TCM diagnosis relies on the four diagnostic methods: observation, listening/smelling, inquiring, and palpation, which gather most of the same information included in the Western clinical file. The four methods also gather information that is not typically included or not given much diagnostic value in the West, but is considered relevant for a correct pattern diagnosis. The most salient examples are observation of the tongue and palpation of the radial pulses, which provide a wealth of qualitative information indispensable to TCM pattern identification.

"Integration of the Four Diagnostic Methods"/Integrate East and West

It must be emphasized that in the practice of TCM, the physician should never rely on one isolated diagnostic method; information from all four methods must be integrated into the diagnosis. Moreover, in the modern clinical practice of Chinese medicine, the value of integrating diagnostic procedures, concepts, and theories from Western biomedicine is becoming increasingly important.

Table 3.2 Clinical record (conventional TCM)

Information	Clinical value/relevance
Patient's personal information	Same as Western medicine
Family medical history	Same as Western medicine
	Evaluates the strength of kidney essence
Lifestyle history	Same as Western medicine
	Correlates habits, lifestyle, diet, emotional and social influences to health
Personal medical history	Same as Western medicine
Present condition	Same as Western medicine
	Basic information for pattern discrimination
Organ system inquiry	Same as Western biomedical body systems classification
	Correspondence with TCM organ systems
Specific TCM information	Valuable/relevant data for a TCM diagnosis (see Table 3.3)
Physical examination	Same as Western medicine
	Some information with special value to TCM, e.g., point and channel palpation, changes in color, temperature, humidity, tension, rigidity, tenderness, etc.
Examination of channels, regions, and points	Only used in TCM diagnosis
Pulse diagnosis	Only used in TCM diagnosis
	Relevant to pattern discrimination
Tongue diagnosis	Only used in TCM diagnosis
	Relevant to pattern discrimination
Analysis of information	From Western biomedical and traditional Chinese perspectives, including integration of complementary findings of each one
Pattern	Exclusive to TCM
Treatment (integrating TCM and Biomedical)	Integrated and according to the needs of the patient
Follow-up	Same for both systems
Referral/interconsultation	Instances requiring specialized diagnosis or treatment beyond the scope of TCM, i.e., specialized or surgical treatments, etc.

The Clinical Record for TCM Diagnosis

Table 3.2 illustrates the most important items of diagnostic information gathered during a TCM examination. It is also a proposal of the kind of organization a patient file may contain to allow for both Western biomedical and Chinese pattern discrimination diagnoses.

Information Relevant to a TCM Diagnosis (TCM-Specific Information)

Table 3.3 lists items that provide valuable information to a TCM pattern diagnosis, but which are not considered as relevant or important in the Western biomedical model. Generally speaking, neither a general practitioner nor a specialist practitioner of Western medicine will find diagnostic clues or information of any value in this data. However, all of this information is invaluable when analyzed in the context of traditional Chinese medical theory. Taken as a whole, the collection of signs and symptoms is interpreted to reveal the underlying pattern of disharmony affecting the patient.

Essential Questions for TCM Pattern Diagnosis

Table 3.4 lists groups of signs and symptoms frequently encountered in the clinical practice and its most common correspondences to TCM patterns. They should always be investigated and considered of relevant importance for diagnosis and treatment in TCM.

Diagnosis and Treatment in the Integrated TCM/Biomedical Clinic

The following is our proposal for a step-by-step description of the process of diagnosis and treatment in an integrated (TCM/biomedical) medicine setting.

1. Gathering information (inquiry, palpation, observation, listening/smelling)
2. Analysis of information from TCM/biomedical perspectives
3. Integration of all clinical manifestations per TCM organ systems theory
4. Visualization (diagrammatic) of etiology, pathophysiology and most probable interorganic relationships
5. Establish a hierarchy of the most probable disease process(es) at work
6. Establish the main TCM pattern of disharmony
7. Establish secondary patterns
8. Correlate all patterns
9. Establish biomedical diagnosis
10. Analyze and interpret correspondences and parallelisms between TCM and biomedical perspectives
11. Design treatment strategies and prescriptions according to pattern discrimination:
    a. Acupuncture point selection and Chinese herb/formula prescription
    b. Complementary/additional TCM treatment modalities (massage, exercise, diet)
    c. Complementary biomedical treatment

Table 3.3 TCM-relevant information

	TCM-relevant information	Remarks
1	Stools/defecation	Frequency, odor, color, consistency, pain; helps to discern patterns of heat, cold, damp, phlegm, deficiency, excess, qi stagnation, etc
2	Urination	Frequency, odor, color, pain; indicates heat, cold, damp patterns
3	Sweat	Presence/absence, amount, time of day when it occurs, subjective sensations of cold or heat, consistency, relation to activity; indicates qi and yin deficiency, cold and heat patterns
4	Thirst	Presence/absence of preference for hot or cold drinks; especially indicative for heat patterns
5	Sleep pattern	Disturbances, dreams, insomnia; indicates heart, liver, kidney-heart, or spleen-heart patterns
6	Menstruation	Frequency, duration, color, amount, and consistency of blood, clots, pain; indicates deficiency, excess, heat or cold, qi and blood stagnation patterns
7	Emotions	TCM recognizes seven emotions (anger, euphoria, worry, sadness, grief, fear, and fright), the presence/prevalence of any one of which is seen as a marker of illness; especially indicative of heart and liver patterns
8	Diet	Regularity and number of meals per day, amount, specific foods eaten; indicative of food stagnation (indigestion), spleen-stomach, or damp-phlegm patterns
9	Sexual life	Frequency, correlation to patient age; indicator of condition of kidney essence
10	Exercise	Relevant in relation to strengthening the vital energy; excess can be linked to spleen and/or kidney damage
11	Pulse palpation	Indicator of the condition of qi and blood in the organ-channel system; fundamental for TCM Pattern discrimination
12	Tongue observation	Indicator of the condition of the internal organs and the nature of diseases; fundamental for TCM pattern discrimination
13	Pain	Nature/quality of pain, location (regional and channel/organ distribution); indicates cold, heat, damp, qi and blood stagnation patterns. Useful for pattern discrimination and treatment
14	Channel observation/palpation	Presence and location of lesions (discoloration, lumps, nodules, abscesses, scars); correlates to the channel/organ system, useful for pattern discrimination and treatment

Table 3.4 Essential questions for TCM pattern diagnosis

Main clinical manifestations	Principal related patterns
Lumbago, heat in palms and feet or cold feet, knee pain, impotence	Kidney deficiency patterns
Depression, irritability, indecision, stubbornness, bitter mouth, costal pain	Liver stagnation/deficiency patterns
Palpitations, anxiety, insomnia	Heart patterns
Abdominal distension, poor appetite, fatigue; Inflammation, loose stools	Spleen/stomach patterns
Cough, phlegm, stuffy nose, sneezing, itchy nose, throat, ears or eyes, thoracic pain or oppression, skin disorders	Lung patterns
Headache (depending on location)	Yang channels, wind, qi and blood dynamic; wind-cold invasion to *taiyang*, liver *yang* hyperactivity
Epigastric pain, hollow sensation in the mouth of the stomach, nausea, vomiting, heartburn, appetite, meal/food preferences	Stomach/spleen
	Stomach qi counter-flowing upward
	Liver-stomach disharmony
Sleep disorders	Heart, liver, kidney, spleen
Fatigue (depending on time of occurrence)	Kidney, spleen syndromes
Thirst (with or without desire for fluids)	Heat, dampness patterns
Dry skin, forgetfulness, hair loss, constipation, numbness of the limbs, tendency to hypotension, loss of eyesight, excessive dreaming, difficulty in sustaining activity/effort, shoulder pain, difficulty raising the arms, back pain	Blood deficiency
Sweat	Lung, heart patterns
	Qi deficiency
	Yin deficiency
Urination	Painful urinary dribbling patterns
	Damp-heat patterns
	Kidney-yin or kidney-yang patterns
Disturbances in menstruation, leucorrhea	Blood patterns (cold, heat, deficiency, stagnation)
	Dampness

12. Schedule subsequent visits
13. Follow-up and evolution of disease process
14. Interconsultation, referral
15. Other specialized diagnostic procedures (lab tests, imaging, etc.)
16. Prognosis

It is important to explain to the patient how crucial their own commitment to their health is in this model, stressing discipline, constancy, and self-responsibility. Depending on the individual patient's condition and needs, maintenance and preventative visits may also be recommended. Medical acupuncturists should conduct themselves according to the basic principles of the patient–physician relationship at all times, i.e., with interest, trust, cordiality, amiability, honesty, clarity, security, and professionalism.

Syndrome, Pattern, and Disease: TCM and Biomedicine

Syndrome

The word "syndrome" comes from the Greek roots "syn-" meaning together and "dramein" meaning to run; i.e., to run together or to go together. Therefore, the word is defined as "a set of signs and symptoms that tend to occur together, and which reflect the presence of a particular disease." A syndrome is the association of several recognizable clinical features, signs and symptoms, or other phenomena that often occur together. The presence of one or more of these features alerts the physician to look for occurrences of the rest in order to confirm or rule out the syndrome in question.

The description of a syndrome includes a number of essential characteristics that, when concurrent, confirm the diagnosis of a condition. Frequently, said characteristics are divided into (a) typical major symptoms and signs that must be present to confirm the diagnosis and (b) minor findings, some or all of which may be absent. Some technical descriptions will specify the minimum number of major and minor findings required to confirm the diagnosis.

TCM Pattern

A pattern of disharmony in TCM is not a fixed entity. Rather than a collection of signs and symptoms that are specifically linked to a condition or disease, the pattern represents a series of functional relationships that become apparent after a process of analysis and interpretation of all findings in a given situation. The TCM pattern is thus a snapshot of the general state of well-being of an individual at a given time. It can be thought of as a dynamic schematic of the individual's constitutional tendencies, physiological processes, and current influences to their state of health, including lifestyle, emotional disposition, diet, the prevailing weather patterns of their locale, etc. The corollary of this is that a pattern of disharmony may not present as a clearly recognizable "disease," rather, it portrays the tendencies that may lead to pathological manifestations, thus allowing the practitioner to construct a holistic, preventative treatment before a disease process is established.

Pattern Discrimination

Pattern discrimination is the process of analyzing the data obtained through the four methods to arrive at a diagnosis concerning the patient's pattern of disharmony, according to TCM theory. Patterns are discerned from the presence and/or absence of given signs and symptoms in combination. This is important because almost any sign or symptom in Chinese medicine can point to more than one pattern of disharmony, depending on what other signs and symptoms occur with it. The sum total of what is and is not present paints a picture of the current stage of the disease process, revealing its etiology, location, and nature. The pathophysiology of the condition is deducted from the reactions (signs and symptoms) manifested by the patient, which may vary as the condition progresses. This model constitutes the foundation for establishing a therapeutic strategy that addresses the specific current condition of the patient, while also considering their basic constitution, inheritance, environment, and current life circumstance. In sum, the TCM pattern of disharmony reflects the essential nature of the disease process at the moment when it is observed.

A TCM pattern of disharmony reflects the essence of the disease at a given point in time.

Disease vs. Pattern

Disease is often defined as the condition opposite to health, i.e., the absence or lack of health. More specifically, the term broadly refers to any condition that impairs normal function. Disease is the name given to an abnormal (medical) condition that affects the body and is associated with specific symptoms and signs. In many cases, the term disease is used interchangeably with disorder and illness. The term disorder in medicine refers to a functional abnormality or disturbance and is often considered a more value-neutral and less stigmatizing term than disease and syndrome. In biomedical terms, "disease" frequently refers to a certain condition, where the nature and regularity are recognized from its causes. Conversely, a TCM pattern focuses on the organism's reaction, not its cause or etiology, although these can usually be deduced from the overall picture of the patient's disharmony.

Disease and Syndrome in Modern Chinese Medical Practice

Generally speaking, both disease and pattern of disharmony are ways of defining nosological entities, i.e., functional and organic disorders that occur in the body. However, disease in this context is a broader category of manifestation, whereas a pattern refers specifically to the underlying pathological mechanisms that bring the disease into being. A disease process can be divided into stages or parts, each of which would correspond to a pattern; therefore, more than one pattern could underlie a given patient's presentation, or the pattern could change as the disease evolves.

In modern Chinese medical practice, practitioners use the concept of disease to refer to conditions with clearly defined etiology, occurrence, pathomechanism, course, and prognosis (e.g., common cold, dysentery, lung abscess, asthma, hypertension, etc.). However, for TCM treatment to be effective, it must address the underlying process, i.e., the pattern of disharmony. At different stages in its development, any given disease may be the result of different patterns. Conversely, any given pattern may manifest itself in more than one disease. In this context, the disease entity represents the complete pathological process, whereas the pattern explains what is going on at any given stage.

As mentioned earlier, TCM practice demands that the pattern of disharmony underlying a disease presentation be determined prior to arriving at a therapeutic principle and corresponding treatment. In the case of a common cold, for example, a TCM practitioner must determine if the underlying pattern is invasion by wind-heat, wind-cold, or a number of other possible patterns. This conclusion will determine which treatment will be used.

The disease name refers to a clearly defined pathological entity.

The pattern explains the underlying disease mechanism of the disease.

TCM Diseases

Historically, TCM has identified a number of nosological entities whose etiology, occurrence, pathomechanism, and course are well-defined and understood. These are also referred to as "diseases" (*bing*), although they do not exactly correspond to diseases as they are known in biomedicine. Examples of these are atrophy disorder (*wei zheng*), wind-stroke (*zhong feng*), painful obstruction (*bi zheng*), malarial disorder (*nüe ji*), Wasting and Thirsting disorder (*xiao ke bing*), and so on. These TCM diseases are also diagnosed and treated according to their underlying pattern of disharmony, which changes as the condition evolves.

Symptom as Disease in TCM

Conversely, TCM regards some isolated symptoms as separate pathological conditions, which are also referred to as diseases (*bing*). Examples of these include headache (*tou tong*), abdominal pain (*fu tong*), insomnia (*shi mian*), dizziness (*xuan yun*), painful urination (*lin zheng*), and chest pain (*xiong tong*). As always within TCM, pattern discrimination determines the treatment [10, 11].

Pattern Discrimination of Biomedical Diseases

Modern biomedical disease entities can also be subjected to pattern discrimination. In fact, this is commonly done in the integrated practice of biomedicine and TCM, both in China and the West. Diseases such as chronic gastritis, diabetes mellitus, essential hypertension, multiple sclerosis, rheumatoid arthritis, endometriosis, depression, coronary heart disease, etc., present with different patterns of disharmony depending on their stage of evolution and the condition of the patient. This allows for a more integrated and individualized approach to diagnosis and treatment, which frequently allows for more effective clinical results.

Pattern Discrimination Determines Treatment (Bian Zheng Lun Zhi)

As previously explained, the diagnostic information obtained by the four methods is analyzed and interpreted to construct an image of the patient's health and pathogenic tendencies (the underlying pattern of disharmony, even if no actual disease is present). This image is what determines a principle for intervention, which in turn suggests to the practitioner which therapeutic tools may cure, alleviate, or prevent disease. Correct pattern discrimination is an indispensable prerequisite to effective treatment of disease in TCM.

"Same Disease, Different Treatments. Different Diseases, Same Treatment" (Tong Bing Yi Zhi, Yi Bing Tong Zhi)

Because any given disease may exhibit different manifestations at different stages, we know the underlying pathogenic process also changes. As the underlying pattern of disharmony of a disease changes, so too must treatment. This is what is meant by the adage "same disease, different treatment." Conversely, certain stages of development of various seemingly unrelated diseases may be caused by the same underlying pattern, which makes it possible to use the same treatment for all of them. This is what is meant by "different diseases, same treatment."

TCM theory postulates that the body has a set number of possible reactions to pathological changes, each of which can lead to a large number of potential manifestations (i.e., diseases) and that the evolution of a pathological condition may cause the body to react in different ways.

For instance, three patients, all diagnosed with type 2 diabetes may, according to TCM, present with three different patterns: yin deficiency with exuberant heat, qi and yin dual deficiency, and kidney yin and yang dual deficiency. Each of these would require different treatment.

Health and Disease as Continuum

In order to better appreciate the potential of TCM's diagnostic tools, it is important to discard the view that health and disease are two opposing static states. Health and disease occur along a continuum, a constantly moving dynamic process of adaptation to situation and circumstance, which can be influenced through treatment that is sensitive to its mutable nature. A patient requesting treatment must be diagnosed in order to determine the pattern of disharmony at work. However, it is understood that once treatment is implemented the pattern can and will change as a result of various influences. Therefore, the practitioner must re-evaluate, diagnose, and adjust the treatment accordingly. At times, the pattern may change so dramatically as to require an entirely different treatment. This is where the adaptability of TCM's therapeutic methods (acupuncture, herbal therapy, diet, bodywork techniques) really shines.

Integrative Approach

Ideally, all cases should be approached with a view toward integration, including comprehensive information gathering followed by the interpretive approach of TCM pattern discrimination, with an open mind to the possibility of further investigation and treatment using the tools of biomedicine. The best of both systems can be applied to the greatest benefit of the patient.

The temptation exists in clinical practice—especially in the treatment of pain—to resort to a more symptomatic approach to alleviating patients' suffering and to lose sight of the larger integrative view in the process. It is important to avoid doing this, regardless of whether one practices biomedicine or TCM, in order to provide specific, long-lasting, curative effects. It is frequent for practitioners of biomedicine to find themselves without a clear diagnosis, even after numerous diagnostic procedures. The approach of the TCM practitioner requires no time-consuming sophisticated procedures, as diagnosis and pattern discrimination can always be performed, allowing suitable integrative treatment to be delivered without delay. We owe it to our patients to be comprehensive and look deeper than the outward manifestation, to examine the functional relationships at work behind the patient's present condition, and to address them with treatment.

Table 3.5 Categories of pattern discrimination in TCM

The eight principles	Foundation for all other categories, describes disharmony in terms of opposites: interior/exterior, hot/cold, full/empty, yin/yang
	Serves as a super-category for all other categories, see below
Qi, blood, and body fluids	Describes disharmony in terms of the vital substances of the body: deficiency, stagnation, and counterflow of *qi*; deficiency, stasis, heat, or loss of blood; deficiency, excess, or pathological transformation of fluids (edema, phlegm)
	Frequently used in combination with the eight principles and *zang-fu* pattern discrimination
The *zang-fu*	Disharmony is ascribed to one or more of the internal organs, mainly used in internal medicine, one of the most frequently used categories
	Frequently used in combination with the eight principles, and *qi*, blood, and body fluid pattern discrimination
The external pathogenic influences	Disharmony is viewed as the result of invasion from one or more of the external influences: wind, cold, dampness, heat, dryness, summer heat, or fire
The *jing-luo* or channel system	Disharmony manifests along the course of one or more of the acupuncture channels; applies mostly to regional external conditions and pain. Can also be due to internal organ damage manifesting along the course of its associated channel
The six stages	Disharmony due to exterior invasion; one of the oldest classifications of disease in TCM. Mainly used in Chinese herbal medicine for diagnosing and treating acute and chronic internal conditions
The four levels	Used primarily for diagnosis and treatment of febrile infectious diseases that begin with invasion of exterior wind/heat
	Very useful for identifying the progression and regression of many diseases
The *sanjiao*	Also used for febrile diseases, usually in combination with the four levels. Mostly used in herbal practice

Models for Pattern Discrimination

Throughout history, scholars of TCM have developed a number of categories for pattern discrimination. These categories, although not wholly exclusive, do represent the evolution of Chinese medicine over the course of its history. As cultural, social, and environmental factors changed the ways people in China became sick, certain aspects of TCM theory became more relevant, and practitioners sought better ways of understanding the specific pathological conditions they observed most frequently. Table 3.5 lists the most important of these categories, all of which are used in modern clinical practice to some degree. As with all other aspects of TCM diagnosis, none of these categories paints the whole picture of a patient's health. It is helpful to think of these categories as different lenses through which a patient's condition can be viewed and are frequently used together to describe complex cases.

> Pattern discrimination is done based on a series of models or categories that highlight different aspects of the condition and its relationship with body function.
>
> In clinical practice, complex patterns are defined through a combination of these categories. These kinds of presentations are very common.
>
> Combined *zang-fu*, eight principles, and *qi*, blood, and body fluid pattern discrimination is most frequently used in clinical practice.
>
> TCM ascribes patterns to the patient condition, rather than making the patient's condition "fit" the pattern.

Patterns Most Frequently Seen in Modern TCM Practice in the West

1. Liver qi stagnation
2. Liver qi stagnation, spleen deficiency
3. Liver/stomach disharmony
4. Insufficiency of liver blood
5. Hyperactivity of liver yang
6. Liver wind stirring internally
7. Liver and kidney yin deficiency
8. Heart spleen dual deficiency
9. Heart and kidney not interacting
10. Spleen qi deficiency
11. Spleen kidney yang deficiency
12. Food stagnation in the stomach and epigastrium
13. Stomach qi counterflowing upward
14. Wind-cold invading the lungs
15. Lung kidney yin deficiency
16. Lung qi and yin deficiency
17. Large intestine damp heat
18. Kidney qi deficiency
19. Kidney yin deficiency
20. Kidney essence deficiency
21. Kidney yin and yang dual deficiency

22. Urinary bladder damp heat
23. Qi and blood deficiency
24. Blood stagnation
25. Phlegm turbidity obstructing the middle

Summary of TCM pattern discrimination

TCM pattern discrimination provides a more holistic approach to diagnosis and treatment. It focuses on determining the functional relationships that give rise to disease.

Pattern discrimination consists of a comprehensive analysis of symptoms and signs, as well as an appreciation for the relative strength of the body's resources against the pathogenic factor(s).

Identification of the underlying pattern of disharmony allows the practitioner to determine nature and location of the disharmony, treatment principle and techniques, as well as a prognosis for the patient.

Symptoms and signs have meaning only in relation to all the others.

Treatment can be tailored to the exact needs and characteristics of each individual patient.

Pattern discrimination can also be employed to identify constitutional tendencies and mild disharmonies in generally healthy individuals, allowing the practitioner to deliver preventative treatment.

TCM Pain Discrimination

TCM frequently associates various specific pathogenic factors, pathological conditions, and patterns to pain development. At the same time, it is possible to support diagnosis and treatment of different patterns and pathological conditions according to the different types or qualities of pain. Moreover, different types of pain itself could be approached and treated differently according to TCM discrimination.

Tables 3.6 through 3.20 summarize the elements of TCM pattern discrimination, according to pain characteristics [12, 13].

Pathogenic Factors and Pain (Table 3.6)

Table 3.6 Discrimination of pain according to different pathogenic factors

Pathogenic factor	Quality of pain	Accompanying symptoms	Main acupoints
Wind	Moving, wandering, erratic or migratory; changing quality; abrupt onset, acute, paroxysmal	Aversion to wind, slight fever, floating pulse	Fengchi, Fengmen, Fengshi, Fengfu, Yifeng, Bafeng, Baxie
Cold	Fixed, sharp, with stiffness	Improved by warmth and movement, aggravated by cold and rest, tight pulse	Guanyuan, Mingmen, Shenshu, Taibai, Ququan, Zusanli
Heat	Feeling of warmth, redness and swelling, difficult movement	Fever, aversion to heat, thirst, irritability, restlessness, rapid pulse	Dazhui, Hegu, Quchi, Yuji, Jing-well, Ying stream, Jiexi, Ranggu, Yanglingquan, Fuyang
Damp	Very localized, does not move; heaviness, numbness; deep, heavy and dull swelling without edema; appears gradually, chronic	Aggravated in damp weather, heaviness, tiredness, especially in the lower part of the body and limbs, slippery pulse	Yinlingquan, Weizhong, Shuifen, Shuidao, Fuliu, Shuiquan, Chize, Pishu, Sanjiaoshu
Qi stagnation	Moving, diffuse, distending, soft	Aggravated by emotional disturbances bowstring pulse	Taichong, Qihai, Gongsun, Neiguan
Blood stasis	Fixed, stabbing, hard, refuses pressure	Symptoms worsen at night, purplish discolorations, purplish tongue, choppy pulse	Xuehai, Geshu, Ququan, Zhongji

Quality of Pain and Pattern Discrimination
(Tables 3.7, 3.8, and 3.9)

Table 3.7 Quality of pain and major pattern correspondences. (Based on data from [1])

Quality of pain	Associated patterns
Sore pain	Deficiency of qi and blood
Distending pain	Qi stagnation
Stabbing pain	Blood stagnation; after-effect of physical trauma
Sharp pain	Acute qi stagnation and blood stasis
Throbbing pain	Hyperactivity of liver yang; toxic heat invasion/accumulation
Burning pain	Invasion of exogenous wind-heat, or internal heat
Colic pain	Invasion of exogenous cold, or cold accumulation, stagnation of qi in the small intestine, gall bladder or uterus; substantial blockage such as stones, sand, stagnant blood or phlegm
Whole-body pain	Excessive factors, such as qi stagnation, blood stasis or accumulation of damp; qi and blood deficiency
Wandering pain	Painful obstruction (*bi zheng*) primarily due to wind invasion; qi stagnation, mostly in the abdomen and chest; closely related to emotional changes
Pain with fixed location	Blood stasis; invasion of exogenous dampness or damp accumulation
Pain with spasm	Invasion of exogenous cold or wind-cold; liver blood deficiency
Pain with a suffocating feeling	Qi stagnation or damp-phlegm accumulation; painful obstruction in the chest; combined qi stagnation and phlegm accumulation
Radiating pain	Qi stagnation and blood stasis; accumulation of stones or sand in the bowels; liver-gallbladder qi stagnation
Pain with contraction	Invasion of exogenous cold; formation of deficiency-cold congelation due to yang deficiency
Pain with heaviness	Invasion of exogenous dampness; damp accumulation
Pain with swelling	Blood stasis following trauma; damp accumulation; toxic heat
Pain that refuses pressure and massage	Excessive factors: qi stagnation, blood stasis, cold accumulation, food stagnation
Pain relieved by pressure and massage	Deficient factors: qi or blood deficiency; yin or yang deficiency
Pain relieved by warmth	Invasion of exogenous cold; formation of deficiency-cold congelation due to yang deficiency
Pain relieved by cold	Invasion of exogenous heat; heat accumulation
Constant pain	Excessive factors
Intermittent pain	Qi, blood, yin or yang deficiency

Table 3.8 Pain quality and most frequent associated patterns. (Based on data from [13])

Quality of pain		Clinical significance/pattern discrimination	Proposed points
Distending pain	Chest, costal region, abdomen	Qi stagnation	Taichong, Yanglingquan, Zhongwan, Neiguan
	Head and eyes	Hyperactive liver yang; liver fire scorching ascending	Taiyang, Fengchi, Yangfu
Stabbing pain		Blood stasis	Geshu, Shangzhong
Cold pain		Excess type: obstruction of collaterals by pathogenic cold	Dazhui (moxa)
		Deficiency type: insufficiency of yang qi	Shenshu, Mingmen (moxa)
Burning pain		Excess: invasion of pathogenic fire to collaterals	Well points (bloodletting)
		Deficiency: exuberant fire of yin deficiency	Shenshu, Zhaohai, Shuiquan
Heavy pain		Dampness encumbering the qi dynamic; headache with sensation of heaviness can be due to hyperactive liver yang	Baihui, Zhiyang, Qihai, Yanglingquan
Sore pain		Invasion of pathogenic damp obstructing the flow of qi and blood; malnutrition of bones and marrow due to kidney deficiency	Shenmai, Houxi, Zhaohai, Mingmen
Colic pain		Excess pathogenic factor obstructing the qi dynamic; cold congelation obstructing the free flow of qi	Taichong, Hegu, Qihai
Hollow pain		Insufficiency of qi, blood, essence and marrow	Pishu, Shenshu, Taibai, Taixi
Hidden pain		Insufficiency of yang qi, essence and blood; malnutrition to the channels of the internal organs	Guanyuan, Mingmen, Pishu, Shenshu
Migrating	Chest, costal region, abdomen	Qi stagnation	Taichong, Zhigou, Qimen
Trespassing pain	Limbs, joints	Wind-Damp painful obstruction	Yanglingquan, Yinglingquan
Fixed pain	Chest, costal region, abdomen	Blood stasis	Geshu, Shangzhong, Sanyinjiao
	Limbs, joints	Damp-cold/damp-heat obstruction; heat accumulation and blood stasis	Yinlingquan, Diji, Xuehai, Kunlun
Pulling pain		Malnutrition to tendinous channels; obstruction to the flow of tendinous muscular	Jinsuo, Xuanzhong

Table 3.9 Patterns associated with various pain types. (Based on data from [3])

Sore (aching) pain (*suan tong*)	Deficiency, damp evil, or cold evil
	Mostly in limbs and trunk
	Liver and kidney deficiency
	Invasion of wind-cold-damp
Distending pain (*zhang tong*)	Impaired qi dynamic
	Liver depression qi stagnation
	Counterflow liver yang; wind-heat contraction
	Phlegm and food collecting internally
	Liver qi assailing the stomach
	Stagnant food accumulation
Hidden (dull) pain (*yin tong*)	Deficiency, especially when relieved by pressure or rubbing yang qi deficiency or depletion of yin and blood that causes failure to nourish the channels
	Spleen-stomach deficiency cold
	Blood deficiency headache
Hollow (empty) pain (*kong tong*)	Deficiency patterns
	Headaches due to depletion of kidney essence
	Qi and blood depletion
Cold pain (*leng tong*)	Cold evil obstructing the network vessels yang qi deficiency
Colic (gripping) pain (*jiao tong*)	Cold evil assailing the interior
	Obstruction by tangible gallstones
	Blood stasis, or phlegm turbidity
Heavy pain (*zhong tong*)	Dampness
Pulling pain (*che tong*)	Sinews (*jin mai*) lacking nourishment
	Liver patterns
	Wind-cold-phlegm or blood stasis obstructing the sinews
Burning (scorching) pain (*zhuo tong*)	Repletion heat or vacuity heat
Migrating (trespassing, scurrying) pain (cuàn tòng)	Impaired qi dynamic
	Wind prevailing
Stabbing pain (cì tòng)	Blood stasis

Most Frequent Patterns of Pain and its Related Therapeutic Principles (Table 3.10)

Table 3.10 Most frequent patterns of pain and its related therapeutic principles

Pattern type pain	Therapeutic principle	Proposed point formula
Cold pathogenic factor in the surface	Warm the channels, disperse cold, relieve pain	Moxibustion
		Hegu, Dazhui
Cold evil in the interior	Warm the middle, disperse cold, relieve pain	Pishu, Zusanli
		Moxibustion
Deficient (vacuous) cold pain	Strengthen the upright (qi), warm the interior, relieve pain	Mingmen, Guanyuan
		Shenshu, Taixi
		Pishu, Taibai
Heat accumulation pain	Clear heat, resolve depression, relieve pain	Quchi, Yanglingquan
		Jiexi
		Xinjian
Qi stagnation pain	Mobilize qi, guide out obstruction, relieve pain	Taichong, Neiguan
		Qihai, Hegu
Blood stasis pain	Unblock the channels, quicken the blood, relieve pain	Gongsun, Neiguan
		Xuehai, Geshu
		Sanyinjiao
Liver qi depression pain	Soothe the liver, regulate qi, relieve pain	Taichong xinjian
		Fuyang, Yanglingquan
		Qimen
Food stagnation stomach duct pain	Scatter food (accumulation), transform stagnation, relieve pain	Neiguan, Zhongwan
		Zusanli
		Liangmen, Tianshu
Wind-cold pain	Eliminate wind, disperse cold, relieve pain	Fengmen, Feishu
		Houxi, Shenmai
Wind-damp pain	Expel wind, disinhibit dampness, relieve pain	Yanglinquan, Yinlingquan
		Zhubin, Jinmen

Location of Pain and Channel Association

Location of the pain can be associated to the acupuncture channels that traverse the region. This can also be used to determine treatment by choosing points along the course of the affected channel, even if they are not at the location of the pain (Table 3.11).

Table 3.11 Location of pain and channel association

Channel	Location
Liver and gallbladder channels	Vertex and/or temporal
	Ear
	Costal region
	Hepatitis
	Cholecystitis
	Lower abdomen
	Inguinal hernia
	Interior aspect of the thigh
	Yin organs
	Eye pain
Heart and small intestine channels	External canthus
	Face
	Chest
	Scapula
	Interior aspect of the arms
	Painful tongue
	True heart pain
	Painful urination
Spleen and stomach channels	Frontal (forehead)
	Upper teeth
	Tongue
	Stomach duct
	Upper abdomen
	Lateral aspect of the legs
Lung and large intestine channels	Nose
	Throat
	Lower teeth
	Shoulder and back
	Chest
	Anus
	Elbow
Kidney and urinary bladder channels	Vertex
	Spine
	Back
	Lumbar region
	Coccyx
	Lower abdomen
	Feet
	Toothache and ear pain

Pattern Discrimination in Common Pain Conditions

1. Headache discrimination (Table 3.12)
2. Chest pain discrimination (Table 3.13)
3. Costal pain (Table 3.14)
4. Stomach pain (Table 3.15)
5. Abdominal pain (Table 3.16)
6. Back pain (Table 3.17)
7. Lumbar pain (Table 3.18)
8. Limbs pain (Table 3.19)
9. Generalized Pain (Table 3.20)

Integrated Pattern Discrimination: TCM and Biomedicine

A growing number of practitioners in China and Western countries use TCM and biomedicine together, both as the main form of treatment and as complementary care.

TCM Pattern Discrimination Using Biomedical Diagnostic Procedures

According to a growing body of research, clear correlations can be drawn between TCM patterns and laboratory tests, as well as with other diagnostic biomedicine procedures. Many clinicians in China integrate these findings to their pattern discrimination process with great success, allowing for better treatment through the use of acupuncture and herbal medicine. For example, in performing pattern discrimination for gastritis, gastric and duodenal ulcer cases, endoscopy findings are of great value to diagnosis process and in identifying an appropriate prescription that corresponds to the TCM pattern.

Integrative Research: TCM for Modern Biomedical Diseases

TCM has proved effective in the treatment of chronic and complex diseases for centuries. Through the incorporation of tools and concepts from biomedical research, such as molecular biology, it has become possible in modern times to study the relationships between biomedically defined diseases and TCM patterns of disharmony. The effects of TCM's therapeutic modalities on various organic systems have also been analyzed from the biomedical perspective, with positive results. Pattern discrimination can be employed side by side with pathophysiological and molecular biology findings to diagnose numerous disorders, including asthma, systemic lupus erythematosus, multiple sclerosis, diabetes mellitus, AIDS, cancer, and various infectious diseases.

3 Pattern Discrimination in Traditional Chinese Medicine (TCM)

Table 3.12 Headache discrimination. (Based on data from [13])

Characteristics	Pattern discrimination	Proposed points
Recent, acute, severe pain	Excess patterns. Obstruction by six external pathogenic factors, phlegm-turbidity, blood stasis or ascending to block the clear orifices (brain, sense organs)	Shenmai, Houxi, Hegu, Neiguan. Yang channels Well points
Chronic pain, slow evolution	Deficiency patterns. Insufficiency of qi, blood, essence; vacuity of the brain orifices	Yin channels Yuan points
Connected to the nape and back, occipital region	Taiyang channel headache	Kunlun, Tianzhu
At the sides, temporal region	Shaoyang channel headache	Zulingqi, Yangzhi, Taiyang, Shuaigu
At the frontal region, forehead	Yangming channel headache	Hegu, Jiexi, Yintang
At the vertex	Juejing channel headache	Taichong, Yangzhi, Baihui

Table 3.13 Chest pain discrimination. (Based on data from [13])

Characteristics	Pattern discrimination	Proposed points
Chest pain occurs when depressed; appears and disappears intermittently	Phlegm and blood stasis obstructing the heart vessels	Neiguan, Shanzhong
Severe chest pain, bluish-dark facial tint, cold limbs	Blockage of heart vessels by blood stasis	Gahuangshu, Geshu
Chest pain, red cheeks, night sweats, afternoon hectic fever	Lung yin deficiency, deficient fire scorches the collaterals	Lieque, Zhongfu, Zhaohai
Chest pain, cough, dyspnea, coarse breathing, high fever, red face	Pathogenic heat accumulated in the lung, inadequate perfusion of lung collaterals	Shanzhong, Yuji
Chest pain, high fever, cough, expectorating foul purulent and bloody sputum	Heat and phlegm obstructing the lung; heat accumulation and blood stasis	Quchi, Chize, Ximen
Local protrusion with no color change, pulling pain along the ribs	Qi stagnation with phlegm and blood stasis	Yanglingquan, Yangfu, Fenglong, Geshu

Table 3.14 Costal pain. (Based on data from [13])

Characteristics	Pattern discrimination	Proposed points
Distending pain, relief when sighing	Liver qi stagnation	Taichong, Qimen
Distending pain, bitter mouth, poor appetite	Damp-heat in the liver and gallbladder	Yanglingquan, Yinlingquan, Gongsun
Burning pain, anxiety and irritability	Exuberant fire in liver and gallbladder	Yangfu, Qiuxu, Shenmen
Dull, hidden pain, course and dry eyes	Liver yin deficiency	Taichong, Ququan, Yinggu
Intercostal bulk, aggravates with cough	Suspended rheum	Yanglingquan, Zhigou

Table 3.15 Stomach pain. (Based on data from [13])

Characteristics	Pattern discrimination	Proposed points
Aggravates after meals	Excess patterns	Neiguan, Shangqiu
Decreases after meals	Deficiency patterns	Zusanli, Taibai
Abrupt pain, pain on pressure, rebound	Stomach perforation	Liangqiu, Liangmen
Irregular pain, persistent, evident weight lost	Consider stomach cancer	Zusanli, Zhongwan, Gongsun

Table 3.16 Abdominal pain. (Based on data from [13])

Characteristics	Pattern discrimination	Proposed points
Pain increases with compression	Excess patterns: cold, heat, qi, blood, food or parasites stagnation	Shanqiu, Zhongwan, Tianshu
Pain relief with compression	Deficiency patterns: qi, blood, yang, yin deficiency	Sanjiyiao, Zusanli, Tianshu
Persistent abdominal pain, periods of exacerbation, abdominal distention, vomit and nausea	Intestinal obstruction	Chongyang, Xiajuxu, Zhongwan, Neiguan
Generalized abdominal pain, pain increases with pressure and sudden decompression (rebound tenderness)	Intestinal perforation, peritonitis, sepsis	Langweixue (appendicitis point), Liangqiu, Fujie
Sudden and severe pain located in the flanks, pelvic or close to navel	Urinary lithiasis	Diji, Shuidao, Jingmen

3 Pattern Discrimination in Traditional Chinese Medicine (TCM)

Table 3.17 Back pain. (Based on data from [13])

Characteristics	Pattern discrimination	Proposed points
Back pain incapable of bend or face upward	Cold and damp stagnation or lesion of dumai channel	Houxi, Shenmai
Back pain that reaches the neck	Wind cold attacks Taiyang channel	Dazhui, Fengmen, Houxi
Back and shoulder pain	Cold and damp stagnation, channel's qi blockage	Fengchi, Dazhu, Jianjing

Table 3.18 Lumbar pain. (Based on data from [13])

Characteristics	Pattern discrimination	Proposed points
Lumbar cold pain, worsens with humidity	Cold and damp stagnation	Kunlun, Sanjiaoshu
Sore pain and weak lumbar area	Kidney deficiency	Zhaohai-Lieque, Shenshu
Severe lumbar pain that irradiates to lower limbs	Collateral's blood stagnation, lumbar vertebra pathology	Dachangshu, Yanglingquan
Lumbar pain that reaches the abdomen	Daimai "Belt Channel" lesion	Zulingqi-Waiguan, Daimai
Intense pain that irradiates to pelvic area, hematuria	Urinary lithiasis	Shuidao, Yinlingquan, Shuiquan, Jingmen

Table 3.19 Limbs pain. (Based on data from [13])

Tendinomuscular and joints pain	Bi syndrome (wind, cold and damp association)	Yanglingquan, Huangdiao
Ankle, leg or knee sore pain	Spleen stomach qi deficiency, Kidney deficiency	Sanyinjiao, Shanqiu, Yingu

Table 3.20 Generalized pain. (Based on data from [13])

Characteristics	Pattern discrimination	Proposed points
Recent disease	Excess patterns: wind, cold, damp invasion or epidemic toxic damp-heat	Dazhui, Shenmai-Houxi
Chronic disease	Deficiency patterns: qi and blood deficiency, lack of proper nutrition	Shenshu, Zhaohai-Lieque

TCM and Molecular Biology

Some of the most exciting findings in integrative TCM–Biomedicine research are those related to molecular biology. It is now known that certain changes at the molecular level, such as the relationship between cAMP and cGMP with autonomous nervous system activity, reflect in what TCM views as patterns of yin and yang deficiency.

Pattern Discrimination at the Molecular Level

Some researchers believe that TCM diagnostic science should avail itself of the advances of modern science at the microscopic level. These researchers are looking at re-evaluating TCM patterns of disharmony at the molecular level. Pattern micro-discrimination uses a combination of modern diagnostic tools and biomolecular indicators, integrated into the TCM diagnostic technique, to arrive at pattern discrimination. This research is aimed at discovering biomolecular indicators for TCM patterns, especially those affecting the spleen and kidney organ systems. These exciting developments could lead to the development of a clinical practice guided by TCM theory and supported by modern science to improve the quality of treatment and clinical results.

References

1. Zhen H, Fei-xia D. Clinical reasoning in Chinese medicine. People's Medical Publishing House; 2008.
2. Peilin S. The treatment of pain with Chinese herbs and acupuncture. Churchill Livingstone; 2002.
3. Zhu-Fan X. Best of traditional Chinese medicine. Beijing: New World Press; 1995.
4. Jianping H. Methodology of traditional Chinese medicine. Beijing: New World Press; 1995.
5. Flaws B, Finney D. A compendium of TCM patterns and treatments. Boulder, CO: Blue Poppy Press Inc.; 1996.
6. Riley D. Treating pain with traditional Chinese medicine. Paradigm Publications; 2003.
7. Maciocia G. Diagnosis in Chinese medicine. A comprehensive guide. Churchill Livingstone; 2004.
8. Fangnan L. Zhongyi zhenghou bianzhi guifan "Chinese medicine pattern differentiation & treatment criteria". Renmin weisheng chubanshe. People's Health Press; 1989.
9. Zhilong Z. Zhengjiu linchuang xuexing jingjie "clinical acupuncture points classification and essential explanations". Renmin weisheng chubanshe. National Health Press; 2009.
10. Fuyi L. Zhongyi zhenduanxue. "Chinese medicine diagnostics" No. 2 Renmin chubanshe. National Press; 2010.
11. Guangxin H, Yanhua Q. Tengtong zhengjiu zhiliaoxue. "Acupuncture therapy for pain" Zhongguo zhongyiyao chubanshe. China's Chinese Medicine Press; 1994.
12. Enjian Z. Zhongyi Zhenghou zhenduan zhiliaoxue. "Chinese medicine diagnostics & syndromatic treatment", Tianjin kexue Jishu chubanshe. Tianjin Science & Technology Press; 1983.
13. Chengyu W. Zhongyi zhenduanxue Yixue Zhukao Koudai Congshu. Chinese medicine diagnostics, easy study test pocket book series Zhongguo Zhongyiyao Chubanshe. China's Chinese Medicine Press; 2004.

Chapter 4
Mechanisms of Acupuncture Analgesia

Annie D. Lee and Eric Shen-Zen Hsu

Introduction

Acupuncture is an effective needling technique from traditional Chinese medicine dating back 3,000 years. Although historically it is been used to treat a variety of different health problems, including obesity, infertility, and colds, it is also commonly used to alleviate pain.

Acupuncture started gaining in popularity and acceptance in the late twentieth century as both a solo and an adjunct therapy for the treatment of pain. By the mid-1990s, support of both physicians and patients to integrate acupuncture into Western medical practice was growing [1]. In November 1997, on the basis of well-designed studies, the National Institute of Health (NIH) supported the use of acupuncture for pain, nausea, vomiting, and post-stroke dysfunction [2]. This increased awareness in the Western community has led to more evidence-based research to clarify the mechanism of acupuncture analgesia. Although there is no one clear pathway, this chapter will review recent literature and scientific theories.

Acupuncture and Traditional Chinese Medicine (TCM)

It is difficult to translate the mechanism of acupuncture analgesia in Western terms, because the philosophy of TCM is entirely different. In brief, TCM believes in the theory of holistic balance between the Yin and Yang and problems arise when there is an imbalance. Acupuncture is used to balance the Yin and Yang, which are

---

E. S.-Z. Hsu (✉)
Pain Management Center, Santa Monica-UCLA Medical Center and Orthopedic Hospital, 1245 16th Street, Suite 225, Santa Monica, California 90404, USA
e-mail: ehsu@mednet.ucla.edu

A. D. Lee
Department of Anesthesiology, University of California at Los Angeles
Los Angeles, USA

manifested to regulate the Qi (energy)and blood. Qi travels through channels called meridians in the body. There are essentially 20 channels with access points, called acupuncture points, strategically aligned along the meridians, which can be manipulated through various techniques to achieve balance of the Qi. These techniques include acupuncture (percutaneous insertion of a fine needle), moxibustion (thermal therapy using the moxa roll herb), acupressure (deep pressure without dermatologic invasion), or electroacupuncture (EA) (electrical stimulation of needles at acupoints). Even with acupuncture alone there are specific techniques of twisting the needle side to side and up and down to capture the Qi. The practitioner often describes this capture, termed De Qi, as a sense of tightness around the needle as it enters deep tissues. In TCM, it is thought of as "the fish taking the bait" when the acupuncture point stimulates the imbalanced Qi. The sensation experienced by the patient is often soreness, numbness, heaviness, or even an electrical sensation. Acupuncture relieves pain and illness by unblocking stagnant Qi in the meridians, thereby restoring the balance between Yin and Yang.

Translating Acupuncture Analgesia in Terms of Western Medicine: Evidence-Based Research

Since the 1970s, there have been a growing number of evidence-based research studies employing a variety of different modalities, ranging from human and animal studies to those using technologically advanced imaging to investigate the mechanism of acupuncture analgesia. Arising theories from current literature describe a neural basis for its effect, involving the peripheral and central pain pathways.

Peripheral Mechanism

Sensory Fibers

One of the first human studies to scientifically investigate the effects of acupuncture was conducted in 1973, and tested the analgesic effects of acupuncture against morphine [3]. Two randomly divided groups of volunteers received either acupuncture at the acupoints for large intestine 4 (LI 4) and stomach 36 (ST 36) or morphine intramuscularly. Although both groups showed an increase of 80–90% in their pain thresholds, researchers found that local anesthetic injection of 2% procaine at LI 4 demolished any acupuncture effect or local sensation. Another study used direct stimulation of peripheral nerve sensory fibers and acupuncture needling. It showed that both raised the pain thresholds of the subjects in a similar manner [4]. This report not only supported the finding that acupuncture raises the pain threshold but also revealed evidence that acupoints may be related to peripheral nerve sensory fibers.

Deep Tissue Nerve Fibers

Clinical and observation studies of the similarities of acupuncture to the peripheral nervous system led to a topographic mapping of acupoints to their afferent nerve fibers. Zhou et al. [5] mapped 12 meridians, including Ren meridian, with its 324 acupoints, and saw that 323 had rich innervations. It was proposed that the effectiveness of acupuncture lies within deep tissue innervations and not superficial skin afferent fibers [6]. Volunteers in a study by Chiang et al. [7] experienced increased pain threshold with needling at acupoint LI 4. Procaine administered to the deep branches of the ulnar nerve and median nerve innervating LI 4 eliminated acupuncture-induced analgesia. However, procaine to the cutaneous branches of the radial nerve innervating LI 4 at the skin did not affect the analgesia. This study suggested that deep tissue innervation and not superficial afferents at the skin level are involved in acupuncture analgesia.

Muscle Tissue

Other studies revealing deep tissue mechanism s of acupuncture were derived from needling technique and achieving the De Qi sensation. Because of the twisting and pulling of the needle in the muscle, one proposed mechanism of acupuncture's analgesic effect focused on the afferent receptors in muscle and other deep tissues. This theory stemmed from small clinical and observational studies. Eleven patients had stimulation of ST 36 and subsequently experienced De Qi sensation and activity on electromyography [8]. However, both were abolished after lumbar epidural, leading researchers to conclude that acupoints had afferent muscle receptor innervation through spinal cord pathways.

Connective Tissue

Another theory to explain De Qi lies within the connective tissue itself. In acupuncture, the sensation of De Qi is described as a "fish taking the bait" and this may be a coupling action of the needle with connective tissues during the winding motion of insertion. Zhang et al. [9] found that stimulation of acupoint ST 36 generated analgesia and degranulation of mast cells. Pain relief was diminished with destruction of mast cells with disodium cromoglycate at the acupoint. Yu et al. [10] found similar results with destruction of the ST 36 collagen fibers with type I collagenase. These studies suggest that mast cells in connective tissues may play a role in acupuncture effectiveness.

Pain Fibers

A and C pain fibers relay sensory information from nociceptors and mechanoreceptors to the first order dorsal root ganglion, and subsequently synapse to second order neurons in the dorsal horn of the spinal cord. The sensory information is then transmitted through the anterolateral system, specifically the spinothalamic tract for pain and temperature, and the dorsal column–medial lemniscus system for mechanosensory input. Animal studies showed increased pain thresholds in both chronically dorsal chordotomized and control subjects, but unilateral ventral section of the spinal cord resulted in decreased effect in the contralateral side [11]. This suggested that the anterolateral system for pain and temperature sensation plays an important role in the acupuncture pathway.

Transmission of pain signals and acupuncture signals both require intact nociceptive afferent receptors. Pan et al. [12] showed that there was no response to pain in rats with receptor inhibition using capsaicin. A and C pain fibers have specifically been implicated as being related to acupoints. Li et al. [13] used Evans blue extravasation technique to map C fibers on rat hind limbs. The area of extravasation was in the distribution of acupoints and meridians. The authors concluded that acupoints were areas with high innervation, particularly with pain fibers.

The range of A-type afferents has been shown to illicit a lower nociceptive response in cat spinal dorsal horn neurons [14]. Specifically, EA can stimulate Aβ-type afferents alone to produce analgesia [15]. A recent study by Leung et al. [16] showed increased analgesia with activation of Aδ-type afferents by acupuncture.

C fibers also appear to play a role in acupuncture analgesia. Degeneration of unmyelinated C fibers using capsaicin showed decreased analgesia when acupuncture was introduced to rats [17]. In cat studies, C fiber activity persisted after termination of stimulation at ST 36 [18]. This may correspond to the clinical sensations of continued acupuncture effect for hours and days after treatment.

Acupuncture also uses the descending inhibitory pathway to enhance analgesia. Particularly, EA modulates the nucleus raphe magnus (NRM) of the descending inhibitory pathway to diminish the sensation of painful stimuli [19]. Liu and Wang found that lidocaine injection to the NRM stopped the antagonistic effect against analgesia produced by acupuncture [20]. This supported the notion that descending inhibitory pathways function to enhance acupuncture analgesia.

Central Mechanism: Molecules and Receptors

Opioids

Opioids, including β-endorphins, enkephalins, and dynorphins, are endogenous peptides that bind to μ-, δ-, and κ-receptors to create analgesia. Studies showed decreased acupuncture analgesia in rats that are opiate receptor deficient [21]. Specifically, Cheng and Pomeranz noted the possibility that different frequencies of EA elicited different mechanisms of analgesia [22]. With inhibition of opioid receptors, subsequent studies concluded that low frequency versus high frequency EA caused activation of different opioid receptors [23–26]. Low frequency (2–15 Hz) may release enkephalin, β-endorphin and endomorphins working on μ- and δ-opioid receptors. High frequency (100 Hz) caused release of dynorphin to κ-opioid receptors on the spinal cord.

However, hyperalgesic rats had analgesic effects through μ- and δ-opioid receptors at both low (10 Hz) and high (100 Hz) frequencies [27]. This is contrary to normal animal models that showed only μ- and δ-opioid receptors effect at low frequency and κ-opioid receptor at high frequency. Overall, acupuncture potentiates opioid release in its analgesic pathway, especially with different EA frequencies.

Cholecystokinin (CCK) Octapeptide

CCK-8 also has a significant role in acupuncture analgesia. Increase in CCK-8 via intrathecal injection in mice yielded less pain control under acupuncture, whereas CCK-8 receptor antagonism showed greater analgesia [28]. CCK-8 production is increased in subjects that do not show antinociceptive effects of acupuncture and decreased in those responding to acupuncture analgesia [29]. This suggested that CCK-8 and its receptor have a role in reducing the effects of acupuncture.

5-Hydroxytryptamine (5-HT)

5-HT, aka serotonin, is a neurotransmitter found in the gastrointestinal tract, platelets, and central nervous system. It helps modulate the sense of emotional well-being and decreases nociceptive pain primarily at the NRM in the brainstem. Dong and Jiang [30] showed increase in 5-HT at the NRM in rats with acupuncture analgesia. Further studies by Chang et al. [31] showed a significant decrease in acupuncture analgesia when 5-HT receptors were blocked. Both 5-HT1a and 5-HT3 antagonists blocked EA analgesia at low and high frequencies but 5-HT2 antagonists enhanced analgesia at high frequency (100 Hz). These studies indicated that acupuncture modulates 5-HT release for antinociceptive effects.

N-methyl-D-aspartic Acid (NMDA) Receptor

Glutamate and its receptors, such as the NMDA receptor, are part of the mechanism in the transmission of painful stimuli. Antagonism of NMDA receptors with agents such as ketamine and nitrous oxide, are known to reduce subjective pain and are common agents used in anesthesia and analgesia. EA reduced the expression of NMDA receptors in rats [32], and NMDA receptor inhibition enhanced the effects of acupuncture analgesia [33]. Research suggests that acupuncture may block NMDA receptor and decrease nociception.

Other Neurotransmitters

There are still various neurotransmitters under investigation. Many, including noradrenalin, γ-amino-butyric acid (GABA), and substance P have been implicated in the mechanism of acupuncture analgesia, but substantial data is lacking and sometimes contradictory. Few studies suggested that angiotensin, somatostatin, arginine vasopressin, and neurotensin may indirectly affect antinociceptive effects of acupuncture. Further studies will be needed to clarify their roles in acupuncture.

Cyclooxygenase-2 (COX-2) in Animal Models of Neuropathy and Inflammation

Recent studies suggested that acupuncture decreased the inflammatory process, thereby reducing pain. Using spinal cord glia, which plays a part in inflammation and neuropathic pain, Sun et al. [34] showed increased acupuncture analgesia when glia metabolism was inhibited. Mice induced with Parkinson's disease had decreased microglial and COX-2 activity with acupuncture [35]. The mechanism of acupuncture analgesia may include reducing inflammation via inhibition of glia cells and COX-2 enzymes.

Lau et al. [36] has shown that acupuncture may inhibit COX-2 in the spinal dorsal horn where COX-2 is upregulated after the development of neuropathic pain following spinal nerve ligation (SNL). After L 5 SNL, the rats were treated either with acupuncture applied to Zusanli (ST 36) and Sanyinjiao (SP 6) bilaterally with or without electrical stimulation (2 Hz, 0.5–1.2 mA) four times over 22 days, and/or celecoxib fed daily. EA had a long-lasting and better analgesic effect than celecoxib in reducing neuropathic hypersensitivity. Though COX-2 expression in the spinal dorsal horn by immunostaining was significantly reduced by acupuncture and celecoxib, the superior analgesic mechanism of acupuncture appears well beyond COX-2 inhibition alone.

Central Mechanism: Neurophysiology and Imaging Study

Research has implicated various areas of the brain activated by acupuncture to produce analgesia. Previous studies used blockage of neurotransmission or implementing lesions to determine areas affected in acupuncture analgesia. Newer imaging studies have further suggested that acupuncture and pain have common central pathways. However, these interactions are complex and are yet to be fully understood.

Older Studies

Different frequencies of EA activate different patterns of central nervous system (CNS) involvement. Lower frequency EA elicit a pathway following the arcuate nucleus, periaqueductal gray (PAG), NRM, and spinal cord [37]. At 100 Hz frequency, the PAG is also involved, but through activation of the parabrachial nucleus [37, 38]. Hence, low and high frequency EA both activate the serotonergic system, but through different mechanisms.

Acupuncture may activate the stress response through the hypothalamic–pituitary–adrenocortical axis, but through a different pathway. Pituitary research has shown that anterior pituitary cells are both activated by noxious stimuli and by EA, but that separate hypothalamic nuclei are involved, particularly the arcuate nucleus and adjacent nuclei in the mediobasal hypothalamus in EA [39]. The same researchers also found increases in adrenocorticotropic hormone (ACTH) and β-endorphin with both stimuli [40]. They concluded that EA activated a stress response via the hypothalamic–pituitary–adrenocortical axis, but with a different mechanism of action at the level of the hypothalamus. Lao et al. [41] saw increased glucocorticoid levels and longer analgesic effects at EA of 10 Hz versus 100 Hz, suggesting stronger and longer-lasting analgesia with low frequency EA.

Functional Resonance Magnetic Imaging (fMRI) Studies

The PAG plays a key role in the gate control theory of pain [42]. It serves to inhibit certain transmissions of nociceptive stimuli before reaching the cognitive areas that process pain. fMRI studies showed activation of the PAG during LI 4 acupuncture [43]. Sham acupuncture resulted in a decrease in PAG activity. Liu et al. concluded that acupuncture increased the inhibitory transmission of painful stimuli at the PAG area leading to decreased awareness of pain.

Acupuncture has been correlated to activity in the hypothalamus, specifically the arcuate nucleus and preoptic area. This includes fMRI studies of manual acupuncture stimulation [44], which also deactivates other areas of the limbic system known to process pain sensation. EA was also seen in fMRI studies to activate areas of the hypothalamus [45]. A follow-up study by Hui et al. [46] more specifically assessed the areas of brain involvement in subjects experiencing De Qi sensation, with and without sharp pain. Again, the hypothalamus, along with other areas of the limbic system, had decreased activity on fMRI. Besides the limbic system, which contributes to processing pain emotion, imaging studies have shown acupuncture-induced changes in other areas during analgesia as well. In a volunteer study, healthy subjects were exposed to cold pain and received either electrical or sham acupuncture [47]. Subjects in the electrical acupuncture group reported less pain and had fMRI imaging showing activity in the somatosensory areas, medial prefrontal and dorsal anterior cingulated cortices. This suggests that acupuncture analgesia may have a role in modulating the emotional and sensory areas that help process pain sensations.

More recent fMRI data showed cortical and subcortical activity with manipulation of acupuncture points compared with sham points. Eighteen healthy subjects without known neurological or psychiatric histories participated in both sham acupuncture and true acupuncture at ST 36 two days later [48]. Sensations related to the De Qi effect were correlated with imaging. A combination of conventional general linear model (GLM) and independent component analysis (ICA) was used to analyze the fMRI images. The De Qi sensation and prolonged acupuncture benefits had statistically significant effects on the anterior cingulated cortex, ventrolateral prefrontal cortex, supplementary motor area, primary and secondary somatosensory cortices, occipital cortices, and the midbrain.

Interestingly, propofol-based anesthesia reduced the cerebral response caused by acupuncture stimulation. fMRI studies of volunteers receiving acupuncture at ST 36, both awake and under anesthesia, in a pair t-test crossover study showed decreased cerebral involvement [49]. There were less blood oxygenation level-dependent signals induced by acupuncture under propofol anesthesia in the thalamus, red nucleus, insula, periductal gray, and auditory areas of the brain. Cerebral depression with propofol interferes with acupuncture's effects on the brain.

More recent research has also suggested a top–down mechanism of acupuncture analgesia. Areas of cognitive processing and emotional evaluation, including the second somatosensory area (SII), insula, dorsomedial prefrontal cortex, posterior cingulate, and precuneus, have been implicated using fMRI [50]. Subjects stimulated at PC 6 acupoint were asked to rate their sensations for real versus sham acupuncture. Imaging studies were correlated with the degree of subjective stimulation. The authors concluded that acupuncture may have a mind–body component directed by somatosensory stimulation.

Positron Emission Tomography (PET) Studies

Current sophisticated technology has allowed further insight into areas of cerebral involvement. Harris et al. [51] used PET imaging to compare traditional acupuncture and sham acupuncture. Patients with fibromyalgia were given either traditional acupuncture or sham acupuncture for eight weeks. PET imaging was done at baseline and on week 4 after eight treatments. The results showed μ-opioid receptor binding in the cingulate, insula, caudate, thalamus, and amygdale in both the short and long terms. These effects were not seen in the sham treatment group. The traditional acupuncture group also experienced less pain associated with the increased long-term μ-opioid receptor binding potential.

Single-photon emission computed tomography (SPECT) and PET showed differences in brain perfusion and glucose metabolism after EA at LI 4 and large intestine 11 (LI 11) compared with baseline [52]. Areas involved include the left middle frontal gyrus, the superior parietal gyrus, the right superior frontal gyrus, and the middle parietal gyrus in the SPECT imaging and left superior medial frontal gyrus, the middle frontal gyrus, and the right superior medial frontal gyrus in PET imaging.

Park et al. [53] used fluorodeoxyglucose positron emission tomography combined computed tomography (FDG PET/CT) to analyze specific areas of brain involvement during acupuncture stimulation of LR 3 and ST 44 as compared with baseline. They found increased glucose metabolism in the left insula, bilateral thalami, superior frontal region of the right frontal lobe, and the inferior frontal region of left frontal lobe. However, the left cingulate and parahippocampal areas had decreased metabolism. They concluded that different areas of the brain during acupuncture are identified using FDG PET/CT imaging.

Clinical Implications

The numerous clinical applications of acupuncture and the selection of acupoints and techniques are beyond the scope of this chapter. However, the mechanism of acupuncture stimulation may have an impact on its effectiveness. Lang et al. [54] evaluated the immediate effects of different forms of acupuncture on thermal, mechanical, and vibratory sensory thresholds by quantitative sensory testing (QST) in 24 healthy volunteers. The heat pain threshold was increased after manual acupuncture on the treated and untreated side was compared with baseline. Low- and high-frequency electrostimulation led to a higher mechanical pain threshold on the treated side compared with baseline and manual acupuncture. The pressure pain threshold was also increased by all forms of acupuncture on both sides, with individual changes from baseline ranging from 25 to 52%.

Schliessbach et al. [55] conducted a blinded, placebo-controlled, crossover study to investigate effects of brief manual and electrical stimulation of acupuncture points LI 4 and LI 11 on pressure pain detection thresholds (PPDT), compared with nonpenetrating sham acupuncture (NPSA). EA produced higher PPDT elevation than manual acupuncture and acupuncture in general showed significantly better analgesic effect than NPSA. These effects seemed to be short lasting (5 min) in the context of only brief acupuncture. The advantage of acupuncture to NPSA provided further evidence for acupuncture-specific analgesic effects. EA induced a significantly greater analgesia and less intense pain during stimulation during a brief needle application, compared with manual acupuncture. With the decrease in pain during the procedure and more effective analgesia, this study showed EA to be preferable to manual stimulation in providing acupuncture analgesia.

EA has more recently been shown to have differing effects when employing low versus high frequency stimulation. Zhou et al. [56] studied the effects of acupuncture on the sympathoexcitatory response in rats. They compared manual acupuncture at 2 Hz with low (0.3–0.5 mA at 2 Hz), medium (0.3–0.5 mA at 40 Hz), and high (0.3–0.5 mA at 100 Hz) frequency EA at pericardium 5–6 (P 5–6), Spleen 36–37 (S 36–37), and heart 6–7 (H 6–7) testing cardiovascular reflexes. The cardiovascular pressor reflex response was inhibited with manual acupuncture and low frequency EA, and no difference was seen with medium or high frequency stimulation. Also, stimulating two acupoints that independently decreased reflex response did not produce an additive effect. This suggests that low frequency acupuncture via manual or electrical stimulation may be adequate for effective acupuncture treatment and that multiple acupoints to obtain the same treatment may not be necessary.

Duration of EA also plays a role in effective acupuncture analgesia. Cold thermal pain thresholds were tested in healthy volunteers by alternating between 2 and 100 Hz at 5 mA for durations of 0, 20, 30, and 40 min. Thirty minutes of EA stimulation resulted in the highest threshold, lasting for at least 60 min. Wang et al. [57] suggested that a 30 min duration was the most effective amount of time for producing acupuncture analgesia.

Summary

Acupuncture is a long-practiced mode of treating pain, based on the traditional Chinese medicine theory of the balance of Yin and Yang. While difficult to translate and poorly understood in Western scientific terms, research over the past few decades has shown correlations between acupuncture and neural pathways, including afferent peripheral nerve transduction and transmission, ascending and descending nerve routes, and central processing in the brain. Animal studies and new imaging techniques have yielded insight into acupuncture analgesia even at the molecular level and shown varying areas of modulation in central nervous system. Despite the lack of a clear consensus about the mechanism of its effect on analgesia, acupuncture has been shown to be beneficial in pain management. Clinical research may guide frequency and duration of EA for more effective and systematic treatment. Further research still needs to be conducted to better elucidate the mechanism of acupuncture analgesia.

References

1. Astin JA, Marie A, Pelletier KR, Hansen E, Haskell WL. A review of the incorporation of complementary and alternative medicine by mainstream physicians. Arch Intern Med. 1998;158:2303–10.
2. NIH Consensus Conference. Acupuncture. JAMA 1998;280:1518–24.
3. Research Group of Acupuncture Anesthesia PMC. The effect of acupuncture on human skin pain threshold. Chin Med J. 1973;3:151–7.
4. Lim T, Loh T, Kranz H, Scott D. Acupuncture—effect on normal subjects. Med J Aust. 1977;1:440–2.
5. Zhou PH, Qian PD, Huang DK, Gu HY, Wang HR. A study of the relationships between the points of the channels and peripheral nerves. National Symposia of Acupuncture-Moxibustion & Acupucture Anesthesia, Beijing; 1972. p. 302.
6. Han JS, Zhou Z, Xuan Y. Acupuncture has an analgesic effect in rabbits. Pain. 1983;15:83–91.
7. Chiang CY, Chang CT, Chu HC, Yang LF. Peripheral afferent pathway for acupuncture analgesia. Sci Sin. 1973;16:210–7.
8. Shen E, Wu WY, Du HJ, Wei JY, Zhu DX. Electromyographic activity produced locally by acupuncture manipulation. Chin Med J. 1973;9:532–5.
9. Zhang D, Ding GH, Shen ZY, Yao W, Zhang ZY, Zhang YQ, Lin JY. Influence of mast cell function on the analgesic effect o acupuncture of "Zusanli" (ST 36) in rats. Acupunct Res. 2007;31:147–52.
10. Yu X, Ding G, Huang H, Lin J, Yao W, Zhan R. Role of collagen fibers in acupuncture analgesia therapy on rats. Connect Tissue Res. 2009;50:110–20.
11. Chiang CY, Liu JY, Chu TH, Pai YH, Chang SC. Studies of spinal ascending pathway for acupuncture analgesia. Sci Sin. 1975;18:651–8.
12. Pan B, Castro-Lopes J, Coimbra A. Chemical sensory deafferentation abolishes hypothalamo-pituitary activation induced by noxious stimulation or electroacupuncture but only decreases that caused by immobilization stress. A c-fos study. Neuroscience. 1997;78:1059–68.
13. Li AH, Zhang JM, Xie YK. Human acupuncture points mapped in rats are associated with excitable muscle/skin-nerve complexes with enriched nerve endings. Brain Res. 2004;1012:154–9.

14. Pomeranz B, Cheng R. Suppression of noxious responses in single neurons of cat spinal cord by electroacupuncture and its reversal by the opiate antagonist naloxone. Exp Neurol. 1979;64:327–41.
15. Chung JM, Fang ZR, Hori Y, Lee KH, Willis WD. Prolonged inhibition of primate spinothalamic tract cells by peripheral nerve stimulation. Pain. 1984;19:259–75.
16. Leung A, Khadivi B, Duann JR, Cho ZH, Yaksh T. The effect of ting point (tendinomuscular meridians) electroacupuncture on thermal pain: a model for studying the neuronal mechanism of acupuncture analgesia. J Altern Complement Med. 2005;11:653–61.
17. Zhu LX, Li CY, Yang B, Ji CF, Li WM. The effect of neonatal capsaicin on acupuncture Analgesia. Acupunct Res. 1990;15:285–91.
18. Wei JY, Chang SC, Feng CC. Activation of unmyelinated muscle afferents by acupuncture or pressure exerted on muscle. Acta Zool Sin. 1978;24:21–8.
19. Liu X. The modulation of cerebral cortex and subcortical nuclei on NRM and their role in acupuncture analgesia. Zhn Ci Yan Jiu. 1996;21:4–11.
20. Liu GJ, Wang S. Effects of nucleus raphe magnus and locus coeroleus in descending modulation of habenula on pain threshold and acupuncture analgesia. Acta Pharmacol Sin. 1988;9:18–22.
21. Peets J, Pomeranz B. CXBK mice deficient in opiate receptors show poor electroacupuncture analgesia. Nature. 1978;273:675–6.
22. Cheng RS, Pomeranz B. Electroacupuncture analgesia could be mediated by at least two pain-relieving mechanisms: endorphin and non-endorphin systems. Life Sci. 1979;25:1957–62.
23. Han J. Acupuncture: neuropeptide release produced by electrical stimulation of different frequencies. Trends Neurosci. 2003;26:17–22.
24. Wang Y, Zhang Y, Wang W, Cao Y, Han JS. Effects of synchronous or asynchronous electroacupuncture stimulation with low versus high frequency on spinal opioid release and tail flick nociception. Exp Neurol. 2005;192:156–62.
25. Han JS, Terenius L. Neurochemical basis of AA. Annu Rev Pharmacol Toxicol. 1982;22:193–220.
26. Han JS. Acupuncture: neuropeptide release produced by electrical stimulation of different frequencies. Trends Neurosci. 2003;26:17–22.
27. Huang C, Hu ZP, Long H, Shi YS, Han JS, Wan Y. Attenuation of mechanical but not thermal hyperalgesia by electroacupuncture with the involvement of opioids in rat model of chronic inflammatory pain. Brain Res Bull. 2004;63:99–103.
28. Huang C, Hua ZP, Jiang SZ, Li HT, Han JS, Wan Y. CCK-8 receptor antagonist L365, 260 potentiates the efficacy to and reverses chronic tolerance to electroacupuncture-induced analgesia in mice. Brain Res Bull. 2007;71:447–51.
29. Zhou Y, Sun YH, Shen JM, Han JS. Increased release of immunoreactive CCK-8 by electroacupuncture and enhancement of electroacupucture analgesia by CCK-B antagonist in rat spinal cord. Neuropeptides. 1993;24:139–44.
30. Dong XW, Jiang ZH. Acupuncture-induced analgesia and increase in monoamine fluorescence intensity in the rat nucleus raphe magnus. Acta Phiol Sin. 1981;33:24–9.
31. Chang FC, Tsai HY, Yu MC, Yi PL, Lin JG. The central serotonergic system mediates the analgesic effect of electroacupuncture on Zusanli (ST 36) acupoints. J Bioed Sci. 2004;11:179–85.
32. Sun RQ, Wang HC, Wan Y, Jing Z, Luo F, Hang JS, Wang Y. Suppression of neuropathic pain by peripheral electrical stimulation in rats: a-opioid receptor and NMDA receptor implicated. Exp Neurol. 2004;187:23–9.
33. Huang C, Li HT, Shi YS, Han JS, Wan Y. Ketamine potentiates the effect of electroacupuncture on mechanical allodynia in a rat model of neuropathic pain. Neurosci Lett. 2004;368:327–31.
34. Sun S, Chen WL, Wang PF, Zhao ZQ, Zhang YQ. Disruption of glial function enhances electroacupuncture analgesia in arthritic rats. Exp Neurol. 2006;198:294–302.
35. Kang JM, Park HJ, Choi YG, Choe IH, Park JH, Kim YS, Lim S. Acupuncture inhibits microglial activation and inflammatory events in the MPTP-induced mouse model. Brain Res. 2007;1131:211–9.

36. Lau WK, Lau YM, Zhang HQ, Wong SC, Bian ZX. Electroacupuncture versus celecoxib for neuropathic pain in rat SNL model. Neuroscience. 2010 Oct 13;170(2):655–61.
37. He L. Involvement of endogenous opioid peptides in acupuncture analgesia. Pain. 1987;31:99–121.
38. Guo HF, Tian JH, Wang Y, Fang YP, Hou Y, Han JS. Brain substrates activated by electro acupuncture of different frequencies (I): comparative study on the expression of oncogen c-fos and genes coding for three opioid peptides. Mol Brain Res. 1996;43:157–66.
39. Pan B, Castro-Lopes J, Coimbra A. Activation of anterior lob corticotrophs by electroacupuncture or noxious stimulation in the anesthetized rate, as shown by colocalization of Fos protein with ACTH and beta-endorphin and increased hormone release. Brain Res Bull. 1996;40:175–82.
40. Pan B, Castro-Lopes J, Coimbra A. Chemical sensory deafferentation abolishes hypothalamic pituitary activation induced by noxious stimulation or electroacupuncture but only decreased that caused by immobilization stress. A c-fos study. Neuroscience. 1997;78:1059–68.
41. Lao L, Zhang RX, Zhang G, Wang X, Berman BM, Ren K. A parametric study of electroacupuncture on persistent hyperalgesia and Fos protein expression in rats. Brain Res. 2004;1020:18–29.
42. Melzack R, Wall P. Pain mechanisms: a new theory. Science. 1965;150(3699);971–79.
43. Liu WC, Feldman SC, Cook DB, Hung DL, Xu T, Kalnin AJ, Komisaruk BR. fMRI study of acupuncture-induced periaqueductal gray activity in humans. Neuroreport. 2004;15:1937–40.
44. Hui KK, Liu J, Makris N, Gollub RL, Chen AJ, Moore CI, Kennedy DN, Rosen BR, Kwong KK. Acupuncture modulates the limbic system and subcortical gray structures of the human brain: evidence from fMRI studies in normal subjects. Hum Brain Mapp. 2000;9:13–25.
45. Chiu JH, Chung MS, Cheng HC, Yeh TC, Hsieh JC, Chang CY, Kuo WY, Cheng H, Ho LT. Different central manifestations in response to electroacupuncture at analgesic and nonanalgesic acupoints in rats: a manganese-enhanced functional magnetic resonance imaging study. Can J Vet Res. 2003;67:94–101.
46. Hui KK, Liu J, Marina O, Napadow V, Haselgrove C, Kwong KK, Kennedy DN, Makris N. The integrated response of the human cerebro-cerebellar and limbic systems to acupuncture stimulation at ST36 as evidenced by fMRI. Neuroimage. 2005;27:479–96.
47. Zhang W, Jin Z, Huang J, Zhang YW, Luo F, Chen AC, Han JS. Modulation of cold pain in human brain by electric acupoint stimulation: evidence from fMRI. Neuroreport. 2003;14:1591–6.
48. Liu P, Zhou G, Zhang Y, Dong M, Qin W, Yan K, Sun J, Liu J, Liang J, Deneen KM von, Liu Y, Tain J. The hybrid GLM-ICA investigation on the neural mechanism of acupoint ST 36: an fMRI study. Neurosci Let. 2010;479:267–71.
49. Wang SM, Constable RT, Tokoglu FS, Weiss DA, Freyle D, Kain ZN. Acupuncture-induced blood oxygenation level-dependent signals in awake and anesthetized volunteers: a pilot study. Anesth Analg. 2007;105:490–506.
50. Napadow V, Dhond RP, Kim J, LaCount L, Vangel M, Harris RE, Kettner N, Park K. Brain encoding of acupuncture sensation—coupling on-line rating with fMRI. Neuroimage. 2009;47(3):1055–65.
51. Harris RE, Zubieta JK, Scott DJ, Napadow V, Gracely RH, Clauw DJ. Traditional Chinese acupuncture and placebo (sham) acupuncture are differentiated by their effects on mu-opioid receptors (MORs). Neuroimage. 2009;47(3):1077–85.
52. An YS, Moon SK, Min IK, Kim DY. Changes in regional cerebral blood flow and glucose metabolism following electroacupuncture at LI 4 and LI 11 in normal volunteers. L Altern Complement Med. 2009;15(10):1075–81.
53. Park MS, Sunwoo YY, Jang KS, Han YM, Kim MW, Maeng LS, Hong YP OJH, Chung YA. Changes in brain FDG metabolism induced by acupuncture in healthy volunteers. Acta Radiol. 2010;51(8):947–52.
54. Lang PM, Stoer J, Schober GM, Audette JF, Irnich D. Bilateral acupuncture analgesia observed by quantitative sensory testing in healthy volunteers. Anesth Analg. 2010 May 1;110(5):1448–56.

55. Schliessbach J, Klift E van der, Arendt-Nielsen L, Curatolo M, Streitberger K. The effect of brief electrical and manual acupuncture stimulation on mechanical experimental pain. Pain Med. 2011 Feb;12(2):268–75.
56. Zhou W, Liang-Wu F, Tjen-A-Looi SC, Li P, Longhurst JC. Afferent mechanisms underlying stimulation modality-related modulation of acupuncture-related cardiovascular responses. J Appl Physiol. 2005;98:872–80.
57. Wang SM, Lin EC, Maranets I, Kain ZN. The impact of asynchronous electroacupuncture stimulation duration on cold thermal pain threshold. Anes Analg. 2009;109(3):932–5.

Chapter 5
Common Acupuncture Practices

Shu-Ming Wang

Introduction

Traditional Chinese acupuncture practice is not limited to the insertion and manipulation of needles. In fact, acupuncture stimulations include a whole host of physical stimuli, both invasive and noninvasive applications to the specific points on the body. The ancient Chinese believed that there was a vital energy "Qi" traveling throughout the body through channels called meridians. The rate of Qi flow or lack of Qi flow affects the body's wellbeing. When there is an irregularity of Qi flow, illness occurs. In order to restore health, the ancient Chinese believed that applying physical stimulations such as moxibustion and/or needles into selected area(s) (acupuncture points) of the body regulates the Qi flow and restores health [1].

Early acupuncture practice can be traced back to the Neolithic age with the use of Bian Shi (flat sharpened stone) [2]. Hieroglyphs and pictographs dating from the Shang Dynasty indicate that both acupuncture and moxibusion were practiced in early 1600–1100 BC [3]. The replacement of stone and bone needles with metal occurred around the second century BC. The earliest record of acupuncture is in Shiji (Records of the Grand Historian). The earliest official Chinese medical textbook describing the practice was compiled between 305–204 BC [4]. Later, acupuncture's use spread from China to adjacent countries such as Korea, Japan, and East Asia. From the Han to the Song Dynasty, there were multiple variations of acupuncture written and practiced. In 1023, Song Renezong (the emperor of Song Dynasty) ordered the production of a bronze statuette depicting the meridians and acupuncture points (Fig. 5.1). After the end of the Song Dynasty, acupuncture was viewed as a technique and its practitioners were viewed as technicians rather than scholars. Acupuncture became less common in the succeeding centuries, supplanted by medications and was frequently considered a less prestigious form of practice [5]. As the result, the practice has shifted from exclusively in palace to lay public.

S.-M. Wang (✉)
Anesthesiology and Perioperative Care, University of California (Irvine),
101 The City Drive South, Bldg #53, Rm 228E, Orange, California 92828, USA
e-mail: shuminw1@uci.edu

Fig. 5.1 The bronze statuette with acupuncture points

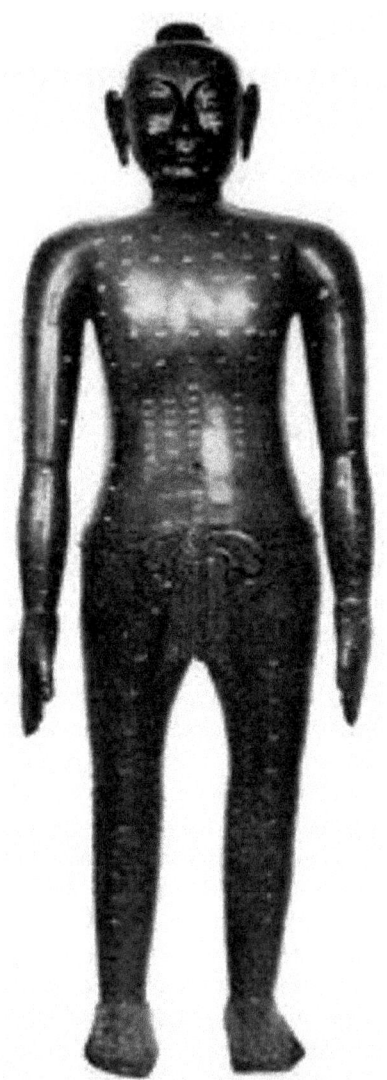

Portuguese missionaries introduced acupuncture to the West in the sixteenth century [6]. Although acupuncture and moxibusion started gaining popularity in Europe, it was declining in China [5]. In 1822, the practice and teaching of acupuncture was banned within the Imperial Academy of Medicine, who deemed it unfit for gentleman-scholars [5]. After 1950 and the Chinese Cultural Revolution, chairman Mao ordered that traditional Chinese medicine, including acupuncture, should once again take the center stage in China's medical practice and acupuncture saw a resurgence in popularity [7]. In 1972, President Nixon visited China, and the visiting delegations watched a conscious patient undergo open-heart surgery performed under acupuncture anesthesia. The Chinese government made a stamp to commemorate

5 Common Acupuncture Practices

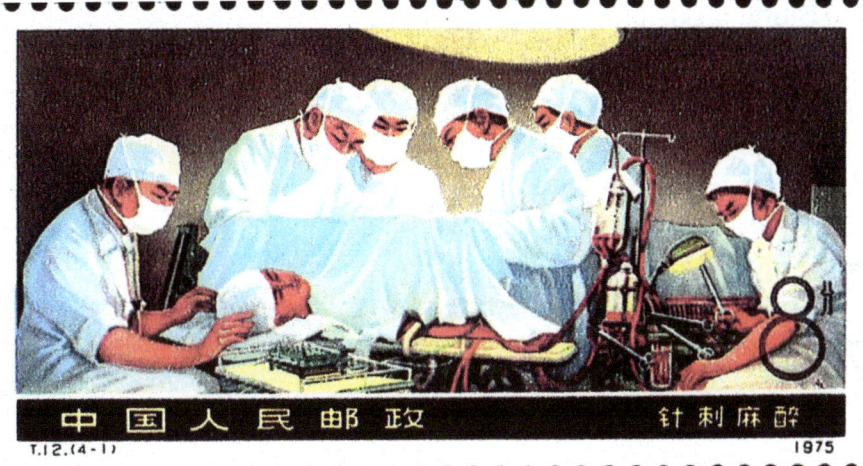

Fig. 5.2 The stamp made to celebrate the success of open heart surgery under acupuncture analgesia

the successful procedure in 1975 (Fig. 5.2) [8]. The New York Times' reporter, James Reston, who had emergency surgery for appendicitis, wrote a front-page article about his experience with acupuncture analgesia for postoperative pain. Since these events, acupuncture has been the subject of active research, including publications regarding acupuncture information and its mechanism of administration [9]. In 1972, the first acupuncture clinic was established in Washington, DC. In 1973, the Internal Revenue Service determined that acupuncture treatment fees may be considered medical deductions [10]. In 1996, the Food and Drug Administration reclassified disposal acupuncture needles from investigational to a class II device, meaning that they have accepted that the devices are safe and effective [11]. In 1999, the National Institutes of Health released a consensus statement indicating that acupuncture is effective for the treatment of nausea and vomiting in adults postoperatively, and as a treatment for chemotherapy patients [1]. However, after more than a decade of clinical trials, the efficacy of acupuncture remains controversial in managing various types of clinical problems [12, 13]. While acupuncture practices are generally becoming more publicized and accepted in the United States, there is still skepticism among general public. Many clinical research studies indicate that the benefit of acupuncture is merely a placebo effect because clinical explanatory trials consistently show a lack of statistical and clinically significant differences in effect between true and sham acupuncture. Although the recent development of non-penetrated needling (placebo needle) (Figs. 5.3 and 5.4) was thought to provide the inert treatment to blind the patient, the treatment outcomes of placebo needles were opposite what the investigators intended. In a research study conducted in a group of orthopedic patients with either acupuncture needles or placebo needles [14], the researchers found that nearly 40 % of subjects reported there were differences in the interventions between these two types of needles. The study results raises concerns with regard to the wholesale adoption of the instrument as a standard form

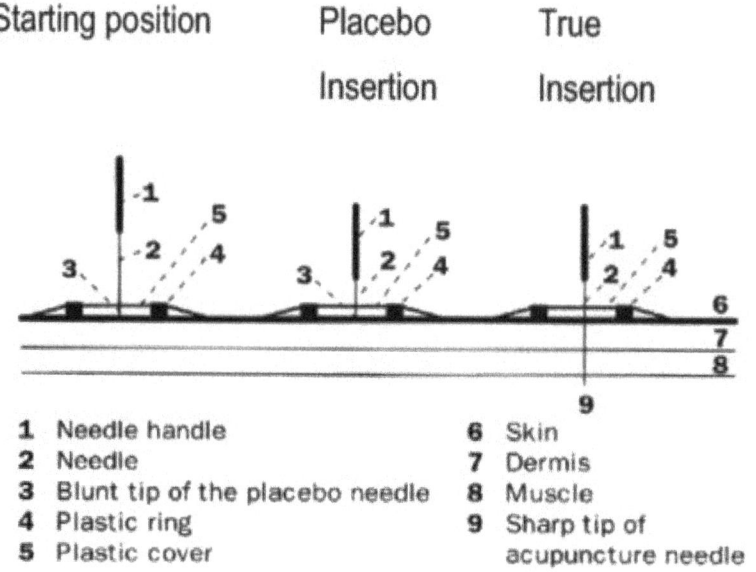

Fig. 5.3 The schematic drawing of placebo acupuncture needle developed by Streitberger [16]

of acupuncture placebo [14]. Thus, the issue of blinding the patients remains. Finally, there is a lack of consensus about what acupuncture actually is. As noted previously, acupuncture practice incorporates different systems, such as body acupuncture and somatotopic microsystem acupuncture, and there are different styles as well, such as Chinese, Japanese, Korean, etc. Different techniques may also be used, such as pressure, needle, moxa, electrical current, laser, cupping, and injection. Many clinical acupuncture trials merely compare two different forms of acupuncture stimulations. It is generally accepted that acupuncture stimulation exerts its effects through the peripheral sensorial receptors. Therefore, any interventions that activate these receptors may produce valid physiological responses. This concept has been overlooked in previous acupuncture clinical trials. The ideal inactive control (placebo) for acupuncture stimulation should not activate any somatosensory activity. While the quest for the ideal placebo control for clinical acupuncture trials continues, the data from both the met-analysis and the pragmatic trials indicate that various acupuncture techniques are cost-effective in several clinical conditions such as low back pain, migraine, osteoarthritis of the knee, etc. [15]. The purpose of this article is not to evaluate the acupuncture clinical trials, but to remind the clinical researchers, physicians, and health care providers that acupuncture is not restricted to penetrating needle manipulations.

5 Common Acupuncture Practices

Fig. 5.4 Each needle assembly comprising an opaque guide tube (*1*) and upper stuffing (*2*) to provide resistance to the needle body during its passage through the guide tube. The body of the penetrating needle (*3*) is longer than the guide tube by an amount equal to the insertion depth. The body of the non-penetrating needle (*4*) is long enough to allow its blunt tip to press against the skin when the needle body is advanced to its limit. The non-penetrating needle contains stuffing in the lower section (*5*) to give a sensation similar to that of skin puncture and tissue penetration. Both needles have a stopped (*6*) that prevents the needles handle (*7*) from advancing further when the sharp tip of the penetrating needle (*9*) reaches the specified position. The pedestal (*10*) on each needle is adhesive, allowing it to adhere firmly to the skin surface, The diameter of the needles used in this study was 0.16 mm [17]

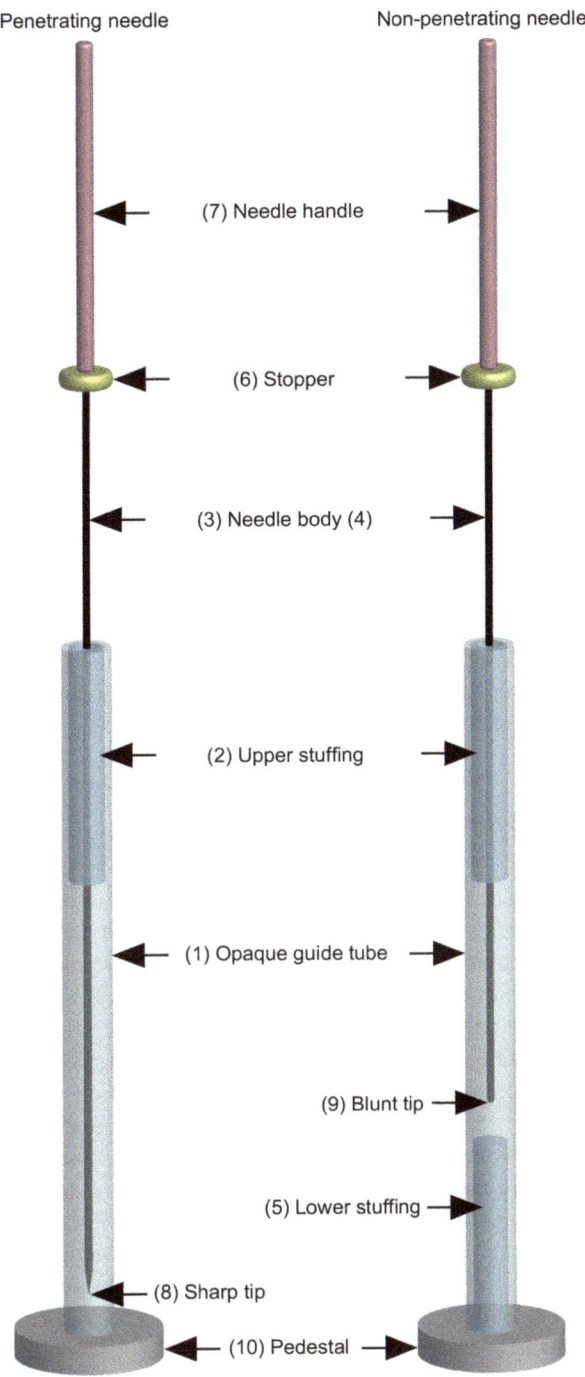

Systems of Acupuncture Practices

Body Acupuncture System

It is the foundation of all current acupuncture practices and is based on the traditional Chinese description of meridians (channels) that connect the internal organs to the skin surface. According to the Chinese acupuncture textbook, there are 14 meridians on the skin's surface. "Qi", vital energy-essence of life, travels along these meridians. When a person is in good health, Qi flows smoothly and regularly, however, when the Qi-flow is disrupted, or flows too quickly or too slowly, illnesses occur. Along these meridians, there are areas (acupuncture points) where Qi runs just below the skin. By applying physical stimulation at these acupuncture points, the disrupted Qi flow can be returned to its normal rhythm and the body is restored to its healthy condition. Chinese classification identifies 361 points along 14 main meridians, however, other points have been identified over time, more than doubling the number of recognized points [18]. Anatomical landmarks and a system of length measurements (cun) are used to determine the locations of acupuncture points [18]. All acupuncture points have empirically determined indications for specific illnesses or problems. Point selection to treat a complaint is typically made after a physical assessment and history is obtained from the patient. The stimulation techniques and durations are determined by the practitioner's interpretation of what is required to restore Qi balance.

Somatotopic Microsystems

It is based on particular somatotopic field comprising of specific points of correspondence (Fig. 5.5). The microsystem was mainly developed in the West and is also commonly known as reflexology. Microsystems are situated on circumscribed parts of the body, such as the hand, ear, nose, scalp, etc. As microsystems resemble cartographies of the organism, they have an allusion to the somatotopic homunculus, as represented at the cerebral hemisphere. Every one of the microsystem points has a clearly defined correlation to and interrelation with a particular organ or function. When there is pathology of an organ or dysfunction, the corresponding reflex point will exhibit pressure allodynia or discoloration, becoming an active reflex point. By applying stimuli to an active reflex point, one can restore the distant pathology or dysfunction back to its normal healthy condition [18, 19]. As a result, microsystem acupuncture is useful in diagnosing and effectively treating illness [20]. The treatment applied to the microsystem can be used alone or in conjunction with the traditional body system to achieve synergistic effects.

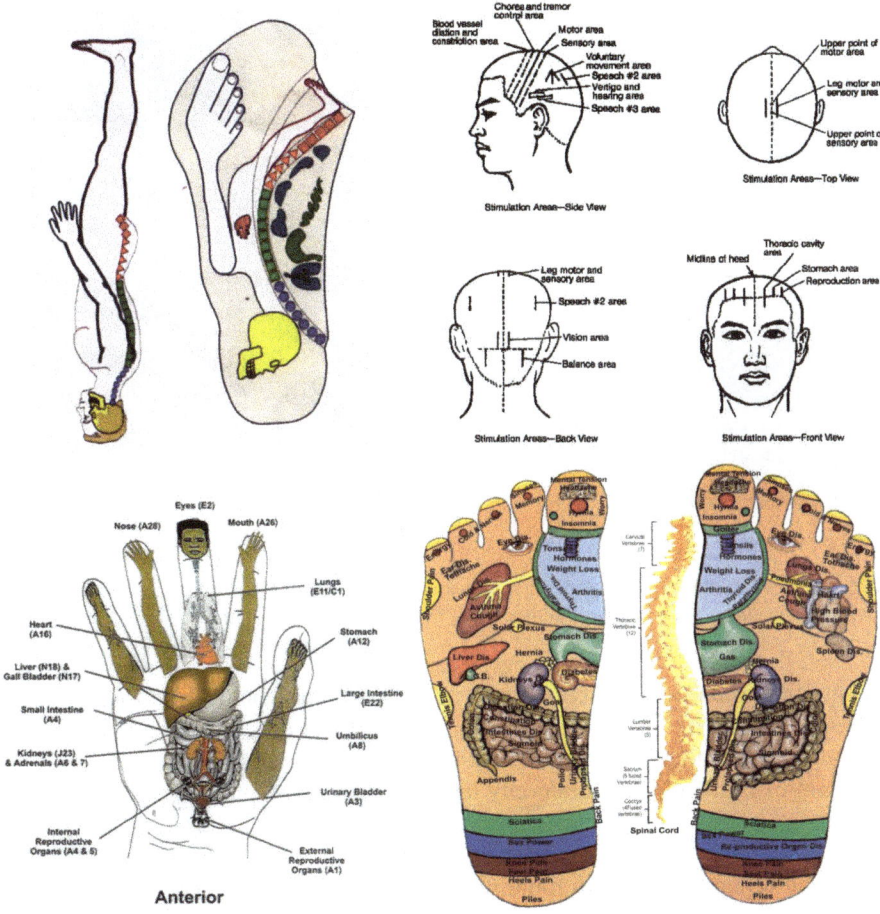

Fig. 5.5 Somatotopic microsystem

Techniques of Stimulation

Direct Pressure

Physical pressure is applied to acupuncture point or reflex point by the hand, elbow, or with various devices (Fig. 5.6). According to the principles of traditional Chinese medicine (TCM), illness occurs when the flow of "Qi" is disturbed. By applying direct pressure to the acupuncture points, one can remove blockages in the meridians and alleviate the Qi's disturbances, thereby restoring health to the body or organ. Tui Na is a form of Chinese pressure therapy, whereby the practitioner uses brushes, kneads, rolls/presses to stimulate the acupuncture points to treat both acute

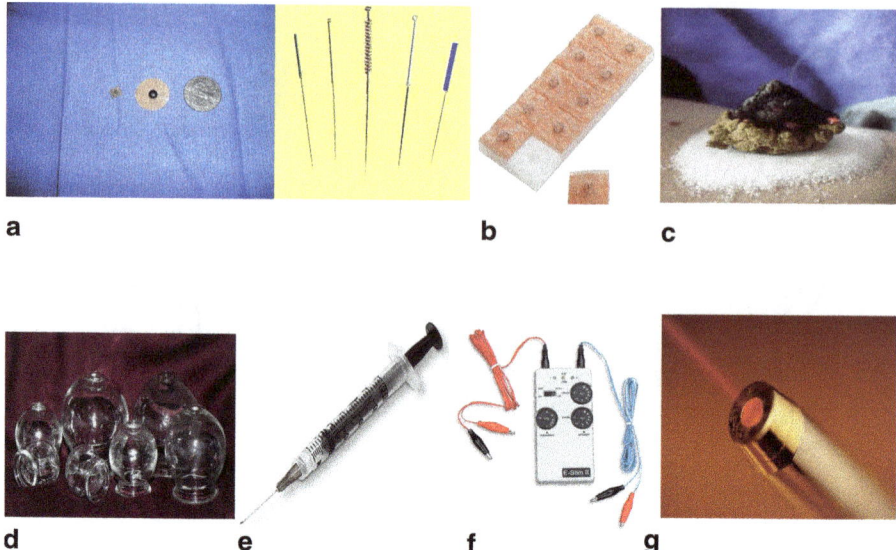

Fig. 5.6 a Acupressure beads. **b** Acupuncture needles and press needles. **c** Moxibustion. **d** Cupping. **e** Syringe and needle for acupoint injection. **f** Electrical stimulator and **g** laser

and chronic musculoskeletal conditions, as well as many nonmusculoskeletal conditions. There are also pressure beads, or magnetic pellets covered with adhesive tape and rollers available commercially that one can apply to the acupuncture point. This form of stimulation is commonly used to treat acute conditions or superficial diseases. In addition, there is the Tapas Acupressure Technique, developed in 1993 by Ms. Tapas Fleming, a California licensed acupuncturist, who claims that the application of light pressure to four areas (the inner corners of both eyes, one-half inch above the space between the eyebrows, and the back of the hand) releases the blockage and allows for healing [21].

Needle

In 1997, the Food and Drug Agency reclassified the acupuncture needle from an investigation device to a class II device. The modern acupuncture needle is constructed of a stainless steel shaft with a handle made of plastic, or spiraled stainless steel, copper, silver, or bronze around one quarter to one half of the needle length [11]. The needles currently used in the United States are solid, hair-thin, sterile, and single-use. Their diameters x length range from 1.2 to 1.6 mm × 15 to 60 mm. Thermoelectric phenomenon has been suggested as one mechanism of needle acupuncture's effectiveness. Scientists believe that when an acupuncture needle is inserted into the skin it creates temperature differences between the tip of the needle and the handle, which directly converts into electric voltage [21]. Another theory is that acupuncture has neurophysiological basis. Professor Pomeranz proposed that the insertion and manipulation of acupuncture needles activate the peripheral nerve fibers, the afferent pathway, and trigger a chain of excitatory and inhibitory responses along the central nervous system [22]. Recently, theories about the connective tissue have been emerging as another mechanism of how acupuncture works. Langevin et al. demonstrated that the insertion and manipulation of acupuncture needles causes the adhesion of fibroblast to the needle, which is known as "de Qi" sensation, a therapeutic signal for both the acupuncturist and the patients [23]. The researchers further suggest that acupuncture needles trigger local connective tissue reorganization [24].

Moxibustion

"Burning of moxa-dried mugwort" is commonly used for any conditions that are considered "deficiency" or stagnation conditions. Moxa is aged mugwort herb grounded to a fluff. When ignited with fire, it generates a lot of smoke. Mugwort is believed to act as an emmenagogue, stimulating blood flow in the pelvic and uterus areas [25]. Traditional acupuncturists believe that moxibustion militates against cold and dampness in the body. Practitioners use moxa to warm regions and acupuncture points with the intention of facilitating the circulation of blood and Qi. The traditional Chinese doctors use this technique either in conjunction with acupuncture needles or alone. When applying burning moxa directly to the acupuncture point, there will be a thin barrier to separate the skin from moxa. The barrier may be a slice of ginger or garlic. Both ginger and garlic are considered to be "warm" herbs, and their combination with moxa is considered to have synergistic effect in replenishing the deficiency or expelling dampness from the body. In China, it is not uncommon for additional herbs to be mixed with moxa to enhance the effect that the practitioner intends to achieve. Finally, owing to the large quantity of smoke generated with the traditional moxibustion, this technique has been replaced by "smokeless" moxa or a heating lamp.

Cupping

This technique involves applying the "vacuum cup" over affected body parts or acupuncture points, with or without acupuncture needles in place [26, 27]. Cupping has been used commonly for hyperactive conditions. When a patient exhibits a hyperactive/excited state, traditional Chinese doctors consider that it stems from a high/rapid flow of Qi in the body. By applying suction cups to the acupuncture points, the excessive energy is drawn out and the Qi-flow returns to a normal rhythm, restoring the patient's health. This particular method is also used to remove toxins from the body and cleanse the Qi. The original cupping technique utilized a bamboo cup. Modern cups are made of glass with a smooth rim. Bruising at the cupping site is the most common adverse effect associated with this form of acupuncture stimulation.

Hydroinjection

This form of stimulation is similar to intramuscular injection. The practitioners use hypodermic needles to deposit fluid or medication into the acupuncture points [28]. According to the practitioners, the dosage of medications needed for the same outcome is less than a systemic intravenous administration and the medication is more effective. It is believed that the medication deposited into the acupuncture points can reach the target organ directly. In China, when young women experience menstrual cramps, Vitamin K3 is deposited into the Spleen 6 acupuncture point to relieve the cramps.

Electrical Stimulation

This is provided by a device that generates continuous electrical pulse to pairs of surface electrodes or pairs of acupuncture needles. There are percutaneous electroacupoint stimulations (PEAS) and electroacupuncture stimulations (EAS). The PEAS is similar to transcutaneous electrical nerve stimulation (TENS). The stimulations are delivered through a device with adjustable intensity and frequency. The major differences between TENS and PEAS are the placements of electrodes and the frequencies and intensity of electrical stimulation. For PEAS, the electrodes are placed on the skin above the traditional acupuncture points, where for TENS, the surface electrodes are placed on the skin along the nerve distribution or adjacent to the affected area [29]. The devices of TENS and PEAS differ in their abilities to adjust the intensity and frequency of electrical stimulations. EAS utilizes the acupuncture needles as electrodes. The needles are inserted into the acupuncture points [30], and once they're in position, a pair of clips attached to a device is connected. EAS has adjustable electrical intensity and frequency. Many experiments have been conducted using this form of stimulations to study acupuncture analgesia. The advantage of these forms of acupuncture stimulation (EAS and PEAS) is that they can be delivered consistently, both in experiments and clinical practice. As a result, researchers have discovered that different frequencies of electrical stimulation trigger different types of opioid peptide releases, either centrally or systemically [31].

Low Intensity Laser and Non-Thermal Laser Irradiation at the Acupuncture Points

This form of stimulation has been clinically applied since the 1970s [32]. The laser was found to be effective as a treatment for postoperative pain and wound infection [33]. The low power laser (LPL) used is also known as "soft" or "cold" laser comprising of three main types: visible red helium–neon laser (HeNe; emitted wavelength of 633 nm), invisible infrared (IR) gallium–arsenide laser (GaAs; emitted wavelength of 904 nm), and gallium–aluminum–aresenide laser (GaAlAs; emitted wavelength of 830 nm). Biomodulatory capacity varies with the wavelengths and types of laser [34]. It is believed that the wavelength for the laser to promote healing should be more than 600 nm. Among these three types of cold laser, HeNe laser may be best for treating wounds and skin ulcers, while GaAs and GaAIAs are more effective for producing analgesia in the deep and superficial tissues. The LPL delivers less than 1 W/m^2. Laser acupuncture relies on the absorption and scattering of light within tissue [35]. Physiological changes caused by lasers include increased phagocytosis, vasodilation, increased rate of regeneration of lymphatic and blood vessels, stimulation of enzyme activity at the wound edges, fibroblast stimulation, keratinocyte and fibrocyte proliferation, scar and keloid reduction, increased ATP and DNA synthesis, and facilitation of the regeneration of muscles, tendons, and nerves. Parameters such as wavelength, output power, radiant power, waveform, and joules delivered per unit area can affect the efficacy of laser acupuncture as treatment for the condition studied [36]. Evidence suggests that the optimal dose for HeNe laser treatment through the skin is between 0.1 and 1 J per acupuncture point. Furthermore, LPL effects become cumulative after repetitive administration.

Adverse Effects

The increasing popularity of acupuncture has led to growing demands for evidence of its effectiveness and safety. Several case-reports and retrospective surveys of practitioners indicate that there are rare adverse events associated with acupuncture, including pneumothorax and hepatitis [37], however, recent prospective studies of adverse events reported by practitioners supports the assertion that "acupuncture is safe in competent hands." When combining two surveys together, over 60,000 consultations were monitored and 86 significant nonserious adverse events were reported, the most common of which were nausea, fainting, and dizziness [38, 39]. MacPherson et al. [40] conducted a nationwide survey, in which patients reported adverse events associated with acupuncture treatment. This prospective survey consists of 9,408 patients who gave consent and 6,348 who completed the 3-month questionnaires. 682 (107/1,000; 95 % CI 100–115) patients reported at least one adverse event over a 3-month period. Three patients reported a serious adverse event. The adverse events were classified into three categories: treatment responses, practitioners' behaviors and equipment, and others. The top five adverse events under each category are presented as follows: severe tiredness and exhaustion, pain at the site of needling, headache or migraine, worsening of symptoms, and severe drowsiness are the major complaints under the category of treatment responses. Needles left in, moxibustion burns, too strong stimulation, especially when using electroacupuncture stimulation, being left unattended in the treatment room, and the breaking of needles are listed under the category of practitioners' behavior and equipment related issues. Lastly, bruising at the needle site, nonspecific aches and pains, emotional/psychological reaction, tiredness/drowsiness, and bleeding at the needle site were also reported by the patients. In summary, while acupuncture treatment is associated with a range of adverse events, serious adverse events were rare.

References

1. NIH Consensus Development Program. Acupuncture-consensus development conference statement. National Institutes of Health: 3–5 Nov 1997.
2. Ma K. The roots and development of Chinese acupuncture: from prehistory to early 20th century. Acupunct Med. 1992;10(Suppl):92–9.
3. Robson T. An introduction to complementary medicine. Sydney: Allen & Unwin; 2004. p. 9.
4. Prioreschi P. A history of medicine. vol. 2. Omaha: Horatius Press; 2004. pp. 147–8.
5. Barnes LL. Needles, herbs, gods, and ghosts: China, healing, and the West to 1848. Cambridge: Harvard University Press; 2005.
6. Dofer L, Moser M, Bahr F, Spindler K, Egarter-Vigl E, Giullén S, Dohr G, Kenner T. A medical report from the stone age? Lancet. 1999;354:1023–5.
7. Crozier RC. Traditional medicine in modern China: science, nationalism, and the tensions of cultural change. Cambridge: Harvard University Press; 1968.
8. Cheng TO. Stamps in cardiology. Acupuncture anaesthesia for open heart surgery. Heart 2000;83:256.
9. Davidson JP. The complete idiot's guide to managing stress. Indianapolis: Alpha Books. 1999; p. 255.
10. Frum D. How we got here: the '70s. New York: Basic Books; 2000. p. 133.
11. Editorial Staff. FDA reclassifies acupuncture needles. Dyn Chiropr. 1996;14(16):1–2.
12. Madsen MV, Gotzsche PC, Hrobjartsson A. Acupuncture treatment for pain: systematic review of randomised clinical trials with acupuncture, placebo acupuncture, and no acupuncture groups. BMJ. 2009;338:a3115.
13. Manheimer E, Linde K, Lao L, Bouter LM, Berman BM. Meta-analysis: acupuncture for osteoarthritis of the knee. Ann Internal Med. 2007;146(12):868–77.
14. White P, Lewith G, Hopwood V, Prescott P. The placebo needle. Is it a valid and convincing placebo for use in acupuncture trials? A randomized, single-blind, cross-over pilot trial. Pain. 2003;106(3):401–9.
15. Cummings M. Modellvorhaben Akupunktur—a summary of the ART, ARC, and GERAC trials. Acupunct Med. 2009;27(1):26–30.
16. Streitberger K, Kleinhenz J. Introducing a placebo needle into acupuncture research. Lancet. 1998;352(9125):364–5. [With permission from Elsevier]
17. Takakura N, Yajima H. Analgesic effect of acupuncture needle penetration: a double-blind crossover study. Open medicine. 2009;3(2):54–61. [With permission from Open Medicine]
18. O'Connor J, Bensky D, editors. Acupuncture: a comprehensive text. Seattle: Eastland Press; 1981.
19. Soliman N, Frank BJ, Nakazawa H, Averil A, Jodorkovsky R. Acupuncture reflex systems of the ear, scalp, and hand. Phys Med Rehabil Cli N Am. 1999;10:547–71.
20. Gleditsch J. Microsystems acupuncture today. In: Hecker HU, Steveling A, Peuker ET, editors. Microsystem acupuncture. New York: Thieme Medical Publisher; 2006.
21. Menzel D. Fundamental formulas of physics. New York: Dover Books; 1990. p. 591.
22. Hsiang-Tung C. Neurophysiological basis of acupuncture analgesia. Sci Sin. 1978;21(6):829–46.
23. Langevin HM, Churchill DL, Cipolla MJ. Mechanical signaling through connective tissue: a mechanism for the therapeutic effect of acupuncture. FASEB. 2001;15:2275–82.
24. Langevin HM, Churchill D, Wu J, Badger GJ, Yandow JA, Fox JR, Krag MH. Evidence of connective tissue involvement in acupuncture. FASEB. 2002;16(8):872–4.
25. Kim JI, Lee MS, Choi TY, Choi SM, Ernst E. Moxibustion for ulcerative colitis: a systematic review and meta-analysis. BMC Gastroenterol. 2010;10:36.
26. Cui J, Zhang G. A survey of thirty years' clinical application of cupping. J Tradit Chin Med. 1989;9(3):151–4.
27. State Administration of Traditional Chinese Medicine and Pharmacy. Advanced textbook on traditional Chinese medicine and pharmacology. Vol. IV. Beijing: New World Press; 1997.

28. Cui JJ, Gao H, Fu WX, Wang YM, Ma SH, Zhang M, Cui HF, Yu XC. A reinforcement of acupuncture on the cardiac effect of dobatamine: exhibition of acupoint's functional specificity. Zhen Ci Yan Jiu. 2010;35(3):188–92.
29. Pinsker MC. Percutaneous electrical nerve stimulation or acupuncture. Response. 1999;89(4):1065.
30. Lytle CD, Thomas BM, Gordon EA, Kraythamer V. Electrostimulators for acupuncture: safety issue. J Altern Complement Med. 2000;6(1):37–44.
31. Han JS. Acupuncture: neuropepetide release produced by electrical stimulation of different frequencies. TRENDS Neurosci. 2003;26(1):17–22.
32. Whittaker P. Laser acupuncture: past, present, and future. Laser Med Sci. 2004;19:69–80.
33. Tsibulyak VN, Lee TS, Alisov AP. Reflexotherapy for analgesia and treatment of infected wounds. Scand J Acup Electrother. 1988;3:137.
34. Kana JS, Hutschenreiter G, Haina D, Waldelich W. Effect of low power density laser radiation on healing of open skin wounds in rats. Arch Surg. 1981;116:293–6.
35. Mester E, Mester AF, Mester A. The biomedical effect of laser application. Lasers Srug Med. 1985;5:31–9.
36. Pöntinen PJ. Low-energy photon therapy. In: Schoen AM, Wynn SG, editors. Complementary and alternate medicine, principles and practice. St. Louis: Mosby; 1998. pp. 247–74.
37. MacPherson H. Fatal and adverse events from acupuncture: allegation, evidence, and implications. J Altern Complement Med. 1999;5(1):47–56.
38. MacPherson H, Thomas KJ, Walters S. Fitter M. The York Acupuncture Safety Study; prospective survey of 34,000 treatment by traditional acupuncturists. BMJ. 2001;323:486–7.
39. White A, Hayoe S, Hart A, Ernst E. Adverse events following acupuncture: prospective survey of 32,000 consultations with doctors and physiotheropists. BMJ. 2001;323:485–6.
40. MacPherson H, Scullion A, Thomas KJ, Walters S. Patient reports of adverse events associated with acupuncture treatment: a prospective national survey. Qual Saf Health Care. 2004;13:349–55.

Chapter 6
Perioperative Acupuncture

Yue-Pang Mok

Introduction

Like many other ancient histories, ancient Chinese history was traditionally written in poetic language to glorify legends. It was not until the last century that Chinese historians began translating the information into documentary formats, with more precision placed on timing and events and employing clearer language. During this transformation, however, and with Chinese history's translation into different languages, some of the original essence, and even some facts, may have been modified.

Major events were frequently summarized in 4–6 sentences in ancient times, allowing modern scholars to use their imaginations to create the rest of the story. Therefore, some of the existing information remains controversial. This phenomenon applies to the history of Chinese medicine and acupuncture development as well. This chapter is based on the author's personal training, research, and understanding. They may differ from other sources.

The clinical efficacy of acupuncture has been demonstrated and proved by modern medical research methodologies. Its scientific merits and physiological phenomenon have been reviewed and assessed through the use of advanced technology. Some of these studies have been described in earlier chapters in this book. They include investigations employing myoneural electrophysiology, radioactive tracer surveyed in imaging, single photon emission computerized tomography, functional magnetic resonance imagining, and neuro-humoral assay. These technologies have confirmed a predictable effect from acupuncture applications, which is also demonstrated by the body's physiological response to the treatment. Acupuncture has not been considered an "investigational procedure" by the U.S. Food and Drug Administration since 1986.

The application of acupuncture in the perioperative setting was not well defined in recorded Chinese history until 60–70 years ago. This chapter reviews its role in preoperative preparation, the intraoperative application of acupuncture assisted anesthesia, and postoperative management of surgical and anesthesia complications.

Y.-P. Mok (✉)
Akron, Ohio, USA
e-mail: ypmok@att.net

This chapter will also introduce the terms "acu-dynamics" and "acu-kinetics", which are the two distinct phenomena observed by the author over his last 30 years as an anesthesiologist. Special emphasis will be placed on the advantage of using acupuncture for analgesia, symptom control, functional maintenance and restoration, reduction of mortality and morbidity, and acceleration of discharge postoperatively.

According to the author's review, there was no clear documentation of a surgical procedure that employed acupuncture application until Han Dynasty in China. The most famous physician in China, Hwa-To, documented the first surgery between 200 BC and 220 AD. Surgeries recorded during that time include the evacuation of a cerebral hematoma, various trauma surgeries for injured warriors, and bowel resection. The documentation describes acupuncture being used intraoperatively, although not specifically in terms of analgesia and anesthesia. Conceptually, it's understandable that acupuncture could reduce pain in most of these cases; however, it takes additional physiological effect to assist in bowel resection in contrast to other procedures.

During the late 1950s, the Chinese government resumed practice of this ancient skill, and placed new emphasis on research and development of acupuncture assisted surgery. The Chinese were eventually successful at reorganizing their information, and achieved significant advances. The term "Acupuncture anesthesia" was coined in the 1970s.

A series of surgical articles were published in China, including papers on craniotomy and thoracotomy performed under acupuncture analgesia-anesthesia. Surgical application of anesthesia was also described in Europe and other Asian countries. The precise timing and events leading up to the introduction of acupuncture application and anesthesia remains controversial, as some procedures were performed without peer-reviewed documentation and publication.

Naturally, acupuncture does not produce "general anesthesia." The patient is usually conscious and somewhat sedated. The surgical site is not rendered completely devoid of sensory function, but pain and discomfort are suppressed significantly enough that the surgical procedure can proceed with no or minimal medication. This chapter will describe the different forms of acupuncture application, in different stages of anesthesia care in coordination with various surgical procedures.

It is vitally important to understand what form of acupuncture one is using. Some are extremely effective at treating chronic pain and disease, but are not applicable to the surgical setting. The most popular schools of acupuncture practiced in the United States include:

1. French Energetic Acupuncture
2. Traditional Chinese Medicine
    a. Ancient Traditional Chinese Medicine
    b. Modern Traditional Chinese Medicine
3. Five Element Acupuncture
4. Japanese Meridian Acupuncture
5. French and Chinese Ear Acupuncture
6. Korean Hand Acupuncture
7. Scalp Acupuncture
8. Other less popular forms of acupuncture

Table 6.1 Numerous approaches for perioperative acupuncture

Acupuncture schools	Symptomatic treatment	Meridian therapy	Constitutional treatment
French energetic	++	+++	++
TCM classical	++	+++	+++
TCM new	++	++	++
Five element	+	++	+++
Japanese	++	+++	++
Auricular	+++	±	+
Hand acupuncture	+++	+++	+++
Scalp acupuncture	+++	±	±
Others	?	?	?

For Western trained physicians, anesthesiologists, and pain management specialists, when using acupuncture clinically, one should be well trained, of course, and skillful in one of these disciplines as a primary means of approach. When applying it for surgical anesthesia, the physician should be familiar with two or three other disciplines as well. They may encounter various limitations in the operating room, which could limit the physician's access to acupuncture points during surgery, and positioning of the patient may also be a factor.

When the anesthesiologist feels proficient in the application of acupuncture, he or she should first try applying it postoperatively for symptomatic relief. Once efficiency in symptomatic control in the postoperative setting is achieved, the physician can attempt it in the intraoperative period. Once the physician is proficient in acupuncture diagnosis, for instance pulse diagnosis, then the preoperative preparation will also become meaningful (Table 6.1).

Pre-operative Preparation

Constitutional Balance

This step is not vital, and the anesthesiologists will often not have time to perform it. The patient may be seen within a week prior to surgery if the condition is appropriate. This preparation might facilitate easier induction of acupuncture treatment during surgery, and is likely to provide a more desirable outcome. Constitutional balance has several forms, but the easiest and the least time consuming to achieve is based on Korean Hand Acupuncture (See Figs. 6.1 and 6.2). This approach utilizes recognition of Yin and Yang pulse. The physician will need specific training in this area to be able to perform it effectively.

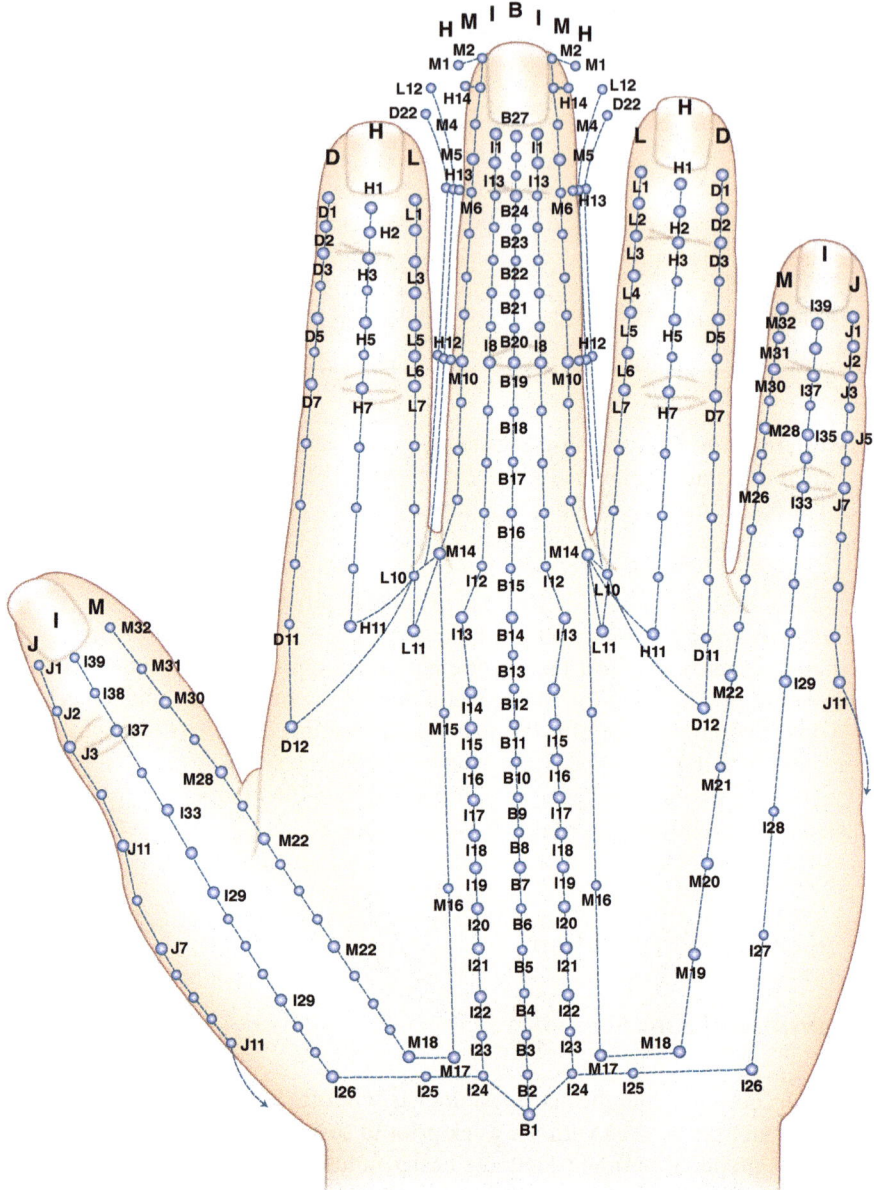

Fig. 6.1. Koryo Hand therapy meridians I

6 Perioperative Acupuncture

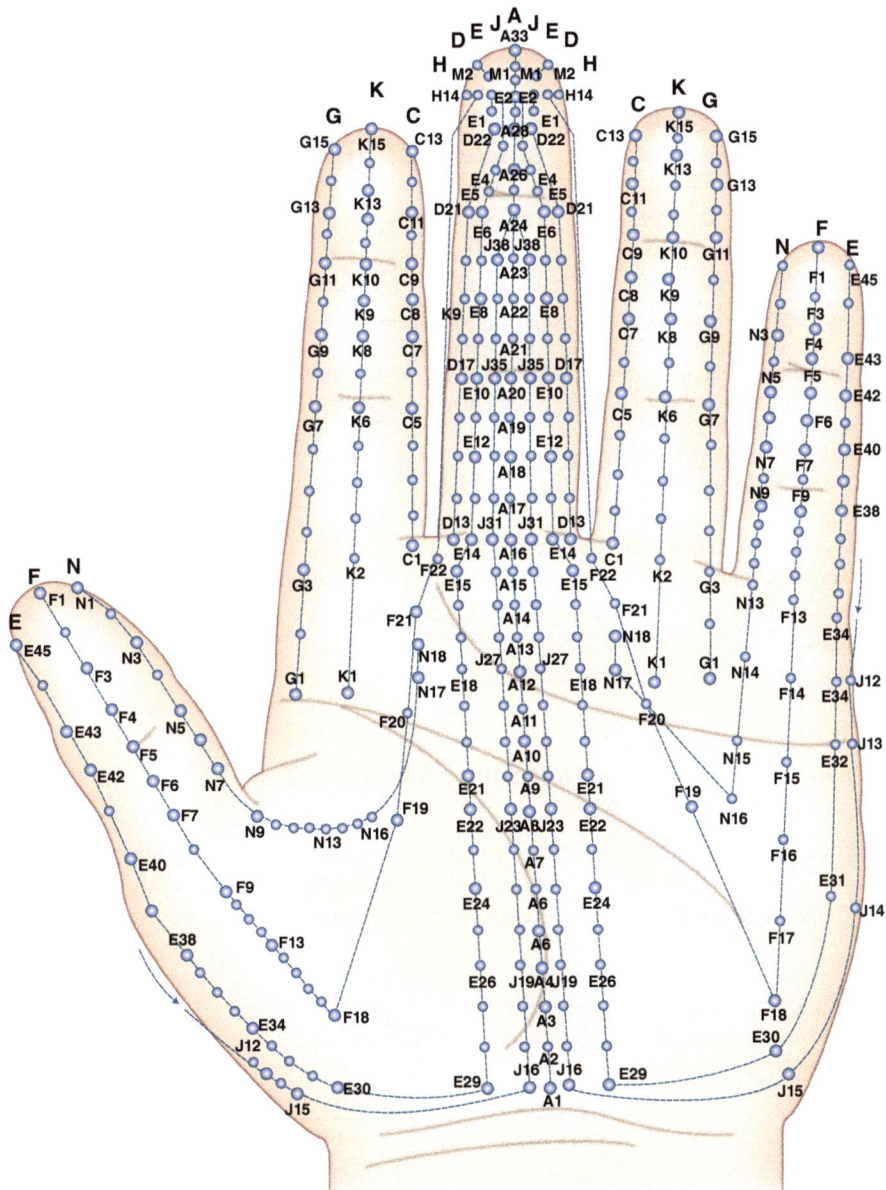

Fig. 6.2. Koryo Hand therapy meridians II

Table 6.2 Yin/Yang pulse (constitutional balance)

	Yang type pulse		Yin type pulse	
Carotid: Radial	Rough	Smooth	Rough	Smooth
4:1	LI sedate or LU tonify	ST sedate or SP tonify	LU sedate or LI tonify	SP sedate or ST tonify
3:1	SI sedate or H tonify	BL sedate or K tonify	H sedate or SI tonify	K sedate or BL tonify
2:1	TE sedate or P tonify	GB sedate or LR tonify	P sedate or TH tonify	LR sedate or GB tonify
1:1	Balanced	Balanced	Balanced	Balanced

TH triple warmer (energizer) (L meridian on hand chart), *PC* pericardium (K meridian on hand chart), *SI* small intestine (H meridian on hand chart), *HI* Heart (G meridian on hand chart), *LI* Large intestine (D meridian on hand chart, *LU* Lung (C meridian on hand chart), *GB* gall bladder (M meridian on hand chart), *LR* liver (N meridian on hand chart), *BL* Urinary bladder (I meridian on hand chart), *KI* kidney (J meridian on hand chart, *ST* stomach (E meridian on hand chart, *SP* spleen (F meridian on hand chart)

Brief description of the general concept:
Yang type pulse = Carotid pulse (ST9) is larger in diameter
Yin type pulse = Radial pulse (LU9) is larger in diameter
Then carotid pulse (ST9)
Treatment based on ratio of pulse diameter (Table 6.2)

Curious Meridians (Extraordinary Meridians)

The constitutional balance and curious meridian treatments are complicated to learn, however, they're very easy to use clinically (Table 6.3). Literally, within 2–3 min, one could complete this part of the preoperative preparation. These procedures do

Table 6.3 Curious meridians in Principle meridians and Korean Hand meridians

	Principle	Korean Hand
	Meridian points	Acupuncture points
	Master coupled	Master coupled
Yang Wei MO	TE5 → GB41	L4 → M31
Dai MO	GB41 → TE5	M31 → L4
Yang Qiao	BL62 → S13	I38 → H2
DU MO	S13 → BL62	H2 → I38
Yin Wei MO	PC6 → SP4	K9 → F4
Chong MO	SP4 → PC6	F4 → K9
Yin Qiao MO	KI6 → LU7	J2 → C8
Ren MO	LU7 → KI6	C8 → J2

enhance later acupuncture treatments, and the same principle is also applicable for the treatment of chronic pain and various internal medicine conditions.

Intra-operative Commonly Used Points

LI4 Contralateral or Bilateral, for Surgeries Above the Clavicles

Sometimes used in chest surgeries in China, this is the Yuan/source point of hand, Yang-Ming [1–5]. LI 4 stimulated endorphin activities govern the front of the head, mouth, teeth, face, and sinuses. LI 4 initiates uterine contraction. It is not to be used in pregnancy until induction of labor if desirable.

Functions	LI 4 regulates Yin and yang, moves Qi and blood
	Disperses wind and calms the spirit
	Clears the meridians and relieves exterior problems
Indications	Relieves pain in head
	Maxillo-facial area
	Fever
	Trismus
	Urticaria
	Induction of uterine contraction

PC-6 "Luo point" of Principle Meridian

"Master point" of Yin Wei Mo.
　"Coupled point" of Chong Mo.

Functions	Calms the heart and spirit
	Balances Yin and Yang
	Cools the three body heaters (Sanjiao) internally
Indications	Mental symptoms of excess fire
	Cardiac arrhythmia and angina pectoris
	Nausea and vomiting
	Hiccups
	Gastrointestinal problems

TE-6 (Zhigou) "Branch Ditch". Fire point. Luo point

Functions Spreads the Qi
　　　　　　Disperses obstruction
　　　　　　Opens the intestines
Indications Shoulder and arm pain
　　　　　　Chest wall pain
　　　　　　Post-thoracotomy
　　　　　　Intercostal neuralgia
　　　　　　Sore throat
　　　　　　Constipation

TE-5 (Waiguan) "Outer gate". Luo point. Master Point of Yang-Wei

Coupled point of Dai-Mo.

Functions Relieves exterior
　　　　　　Disperses heat
　　　　　　Facilitates Qi circulation
Indications High fever
　　　　　　Chest and neck inflammatory conditions
　　　　　　Tinnitus
　　　　　　Migraines
　　　　　　Enuresis
　　　　　　Upper extremity joint pain

LR-3. (Tai-Chong) "Great Pouring". Shu Point. Source Point

Functions	Pacifying the liver
	Extinguishing liver fire
	Bring down rebellious Qi
	Reviving blood
	Discharging damp-heat and perverted wind
Indications	Headaches
	Vertigo
	Hypertension
	Insomnia
	Hepatitis
	Mastitis
	Thrombocytopenia
	Irregular menstruation
	Chest wall pain
	Urinary retention

ST 36. (Zusanli) "Three Miles Point on the Leg". He/Earth Point. Special Command Point for Stomach (Strengthening)

Functions	Governs Sp and St
	Regulates Qi and blood
Indications	Gastroenteritis
	Pancreatitis
	Digestive disorder
	Shock
	Weakness
	Fatigue
	Allergies
	Constipation or diarrhea
	Lower abdominal distention
	Breast diseases
	Nausea/Vomiting

SP 6 (Sanyingjiao) "Three Yin Junction")

Functions	Strengthens the spleen
	Transforms dampness
	Spread the liver Qi
	Nourishes the kidneys
Indications	Abdominal distension
	Borborymus
	Diarrhea
	GYN disorder
	Urinary retention and incontinence
	Sexual dysfunction
	Eczema
	Urticaria

Ear Points (Pain Control Related)

a. Master Point 1-Shen-Men.
b. Master Point 2-Sympathetic.
c. Master Point 3-Thalamus.
Subcortical. Pain Control Point.
d. Master Point 7-Tranquilizer point.
e. Anatomical corresponding points.
f. Lung Point-for skin incision.
g. "Zero point".

KHT ("Hand points".)—"Korean Hand Therapy"

a. Corresponding points.
b. Constitutional balance.
c. Curious meridians.

Scalp points

Midline, between GV20 to GV22 for skin incision.
　General Introduction to Points Combination for surgical analgesia (considering avoidance to contaminate the surgical site; [2, 5–11]).

6 Perioperative Acupuncture

I. *Skin incision*
    LI 4–LI 11
    Auricular   Lung point
                                                                 Shenman

    (Scalp points between GV20 through 22
    Needs 20–30 min electrical stimulation at 2–4 Hz

II. *Oral, facial (procedures above the clavicle)*
    LI 4, ST 44, PC 6
    Auricular   Tranquilizer
                                                                 Thalamus
                                                                 Corresponding points

III. *Chest wall procedures*
    LI 11, TE 5 or 6, ST 41 or 44
    Auricular   Tranquilizer
                                                                 Thalamus
                                                                 Corresponding points

IV. *Intra-thoracic procedures*
    LI 11, TE 6, PC 6, (CV-17, GV-14)
    Auricular   Sympathetic
                                                                 Heart
                                                                 Lung

V. *Upper abdominal procedures*
    LI 11, ST 36, (SP 6 ?) PC 6
    Auricular   Sympathetic
                                                                 Stomach
                                                                 Heart
                                                                 Corresponding

VI. *Pelvic procedures/inguinal, herniorrhaphy*
    LI 11, ST 36, SP 10, PC 6, Dai-Mo
    Auricular   Pelvis
                                                                 Sympathetic
                                                                 Corresponding points

VII. *Genital-rectal procedures*
    LU 6, SI 7, SP 6, LR 1. 2, KI 6
    Auricular   Sympathetic
                                                                 Heart

VIII. *Upper extremities*
    LI 4, TE 5, PC 6, GB 21 and GB 34
    Auricular   Kidney
                                                                 Lung
                                                                 Spleen
                                                                 Corresponding

IX. Lower extremities
     LI 11, ST 36, GB 34, KI 3, LR 3
     Auricular   KI
                                                    LU
                                                    SP
                                                    Corresponding

X.   Obstetrical [12–16]
     1. Hyperemesis gravida
         PC 6, ST 36 (40?), LR 3
         Auricular   LR
                                                    ST
                                                    Sympathetic
                                                    (Shenman?)
         KHT   Spleen jung bang
                                                    Lung jung bang
                                                    Gallbladder jung bang
                                                    Heart sung bang
                                                    Middle and upper
                                                       jiao sedation (KA-
                                                       8,12,16,18,KK-9.
                                                       KF-5)
     2. Conversion of breech position of fetus
         Moxibusiton BL 67
         KHT   KA-1, 3, 5, 6, 8
                                                    KI-19, KT-23. KF-5
     3. Induction of labor (or abortion)
         LI4. SP 6
     4. Labor (the author prefers epidural anesthesia)
         BL 23, BL 26, BL 30, BL 33
         Sp6, LI 4, PC 6.
         Chong Mo. Dai Mo
XI. Other systems used intraoperatively
     1. Nasal, facial, scalp and
         "Barefoot doctor's anesthesia points"

Naturally one must consider anatomical site of the incision, and also avoid interfering with the aseptic sites of the surgeon's work. The general principle is to apply points that enhance endogenous opioid activities. This should be done at least 20–30 min prior to surgery, with low frequency electrical stimulations (1-2 Hz) applied to the needles. The second principle is for an incision next to the auricular point of the lungs, and the midline's skull point. One could apply a pair of needles to each side of the incision, approximately one-half inch from the proposed incision line, and apply high frequency stimulation at 400–1,000 Hz, with a gradual increase in intensity to produce a local anesthetic effect by blocking the A-delta incisional pain. Endorphins stimulation does not completely block A-delta type pain, however, one might also consider applying a local anesthetic.

Postoperative Acupuncture

At this point, I would like to explore a few postoperative considerations other than symptom control [1–5, 17–20]. Acupuncture application in anesthesia procedures is in some ways similar to conventional anesthesia. The anesthetist applies his knowledge and skill to render the patient in a sedated or unconscious state, insensitive to the pain of incision and manipulation, so the surgeon can safely complete the operation. Postoperatively, the anesthetist should reverse the anesthesia and bring the patient back to full consciousness, while providing postoperative symptomatic control. While it is not as measurable and obvious in acupuncture applications, we use the technique to produce a similar anesthetic effect. Therefore, the acupuncture anesthetist should also consider reversing some of this effect, prior to discharging the patient.

In order to achieve this, one could consider acudynamics and acukinetics, in contrast to pharmacokinetics and pharmacodynamics. The oversimplified description of acudynamics is the consideration of how certain points and point combinations will produce predictable physiological effects on the patient's system. Acukinetics is the consideration of how the patient will resist this type of stimulation, how the body processes such effects, and how the body will eventually restore to its optimized condition. The physician should be familiar with this concept to understand why the same point application will produce different effects on different individuals, even contrary to what is taught in acupuncture books

Conclusion

Over the past 25 years, since we first reported our experiences using acupuncture for surgical analgesia, our techniques and philosophy have been further refined.

Acupuncture complimenting medications has many obvious advantages in preoperative preparation for patients with coexisting diseases. This is especially evident in patients with chronic cardiopulmonary diseases. Acupuncture treatment can alleviate chronic symptoms and enhance response to long-term medications in a short period of time. This effect frequently carries through the intraoperative and postoperative periods, helping to facilitate recovery and early discharge.

Acupuncture assisted anesthesia in the intraoperative setting is recommended to bypass the disadvantages of incomplete pain blocking achieved by acupuncture alone. Acupuncture enhances the results of regional and local anesthesia, allowing for a reduction in dose of the intravenous opioids and sedatives given during surgery, or the general anesthetics required. With the modern anesthesia depth-monitoring devices currently available, we should be able to further explore the impact acupuncture can have on general anesthesia.

During the immediate preoperative period, application of acupuncture has been simplified over the years. No more than one to four body points, and/or up to four auricular points are now used. The duration of stimulation with direct current has been reduced to 20 min.

During surgery, some body point needles may be removed if they are interfering with the surgical site, as may auricular points in facial surgeries. Electrical stimulation is only used at points accessible to the anesthesiologist. Additional points may also be added through Microsystems (eg: KHT—hand points, scalp points, and auricular points). The number of needles should be kept to a minimum. Continuous electrical stimulation, especially high frequency and over 30 min, should be avoided.

Postoperatively, treatment of expected and unexpected symptoms may be effectively achieved through the proper use of acupuncture alone, or in conjunction with medications. However, with both preoperative and postoperative use of acupuncture, one should have a thorough understanding of acupuncture theory and rational point combinations in order to achieve the best effect. According to eastern philosophy, acupuncture is used to bring the internal universe (body physiology) to a neutral, harmonious, and balanced state, to adapt to the external universe around us, and to synchronize with the five elements' movements, so one might survive and maintain health. It is not to create a super being with boosted strength, or any abnormal state from what we are meant to be. Formulated "cook-book" approaches, without proper pulse, tongue, and abdominal diagnoses and individualized prescriptions will yield less than satisfactory results.

Intraoperatively, we are going against the philosophy of bringing the body to neutral. We are trying to create an abnormal state of insensitivity to pain, and to reduce awareness and concern (sedation). Although the purpose is noble, we should keep this maneuver to a minimum, and bear in mind our oath as physicians—"Do No Harm."

References

1. Helms JM. Acupuncture energetics: a clinical approach for physicians. Berkeley: Medical Acupuncture Publishers; 1994.
2. Hsueh CC, O'Connor J: Acupuncture a comprehensive text, Shangai College of Traditional Medicine. Seattle: Eastland Press; 1981.
3. Deng L, et. al. Chinese acupuncture and moxibustion. Bejing: Foreign Language Press; 1987.
4. Stux G, Pameranz B. Basics of acupuncture: textbook and atlas. Berlin: Springer-Verlag; 1987.
5. Mok YP. Acupuncture-assisted anesthesia. Med Acupunct. 2001;12 Suppl 1:28–31.
6. Mok YP. Medical acupuncture applications in surgical anesthesia. Med Acupunct. 1993 Suppl 1:20–4.
7. Yang M. Principles and clinical application of acupuncture anesthesia. Hong Kong: Era Book Company; 1986.
9. Liu W. Acupuncture anesthesia: a case report. JAMA. 1972;221 Suppl 1:87–8.
10. Chen T, Chiu Y. A Clinical observation for the posterior atlanto-axial arthrodesis under acupuncture anesthesia. [Chinese] Acupunct Res. 1996;21 Suppl 1:8–10.

11. Chen T, Chiu Y. Normalization of acupuncture anesthesia used in the operation of neoplasm in functional area or deep site of the brain. [Chinese] Acupunct Res. 1996,21 Suppl 1:4–7.
12. Chen T, Chiu Y. Research of clinic and laboratory of face acupuncture effect and the exploration of their afferent pathways. [Chinese] Acupunct Res. 1996,21 Suppl 1:39–44.
13. Tempfer C, Zeisler H, Heinzl H, et al. Influence of acupuncture on maternal serum levels of interleukin-8, prostaglandin F2a, and beta-endorphin: a matched pair study. Obstet Gynecol. 1998;92:245–8.
14. Tsuei JJ, Lai Y, Sharma SD. The Influence of acupuncture stimulation during pregnancy: the induction and inhibition of labor. Obstet Gynecol. 1977;50:479–80.
15. Belluomini J, Litt RC, Lee KA, Katz M. Acupressure for nausea and vomiting of pregnancy: a randomized, blinded study. Obstet Gynecol. 1994;8:245–8.
16. Dundee JW, Sourial FBR, Ghaly RG, Bell PF. P6 acupressure reduces morning sickness. J R Soc Med. 1988;81:456–7.
17. Ghaly RG, Fitzpatrick KT, Dundee JW. Antiemetic studies with traditional Chinese acupuncture: a comparision of manual needling with electrical stimulation and commonly used antiemetics. Anesthesia. 1987;42 Suppl 10:1108–13.
18. Wang B, Tang J, White PF, Naruse R, Sloninsky A, Karinger R, Gold J, Wender RH. Effect of the intensity of transcutaneous acupoint electirical stimulation on the postoperative analgesic requirement. Anesth Analg. 1997;85 Suppl 2:406–13.
19. Ho RT, Jawan B, Fung ST, Cheung HK, Lee JH. Electro-acupuncture and postoperative emesis. Anesthesia. 1990;45 Suppl 4:327–9.
20. Oleson TD. Auriculotherapy manual: Chinese & Western systems of ear acupuncture. Los Angeles: Health Care Alternatives; 1996.
21. Yoo TW. Koryo hand acupuncture. 2nd rev ed. Seoul: Eum Yang Mek Jin Publishing Co; 2001.

Chapter 7
Acupuncture Pain Research: Quantitative and Qualitative

Tat Leang Lee and Zhen Zheng

Introduction

Pain is a major motivating factor for individuals seeking healthcare; however, treatment for many chronic conditions remains unsatisfactory. The initiation of pharmacotherapy and other interventions is largely empiric, due to the lack of a specific mechanism-based diagnosis for chronic pain. Despite significant investment in pain research, the challenges facing the development of novel therapeutics remain significant [1]. Acupuncture and related techniques (see Chap. 5) have been widely used to treat different types of pain conditions, supported by the fact that 41 % of the 3,975 acupuncture research articles published from 1991 to 2009 are related to pain and analgesia [2].

Although there is good evidence in support of acupuncture induced analgesia and mechanistic model of pain from animal studies (see Chap. 4), similar evidence in humans has been lacking. The impetus for a recent surge in acupuncture research can be attributed to the 1997 National Institutes of Health (NIH) Consensus Development Conference on Acupuncture. The meeting concluded that there is sufficient evidence of acupuncture's efficacy to expand its use into conventional medicine, and to encourage further studies of its physiological and clinical value [3]. The formation of the Society for Acupuncture Research has also helped promote and propose strategies to advance research into Oriental medicine systems, which also include acupuncture [4].

Most of the clinical studies performed on acupuncture over the past three decades have been quantitative research, including efficacy and effectiveness trials.

T. L. Lee (✉)
Anaesthesia and Acupuncture Service, National University of Singapore,
National University Hospital, 5 Lower Kent Ridge Road, 119074 Singapore
e-mail: analeetl@nus.edu.sg
e-mail: analeetl@gmail.com

Z. Zheng
Traditional and complementary medicine research program,
Health Innovations Research Institute & School of Health Sciences,
RMIT University, Bundoora, Victoria, Australia

Emergent research strategies include qualitative research. In the quantitative research, deductive approaches are employed to generate hypotheses and data is then collected to test the hypotheses. An example of a question asked during a typical deductive approach is, "how effective is acupuncture in the treatment of chronic low back pain (cLBP), as compared with pharmacotherapy?" The primary outcome measure is the severity of low back pain. In qualitative research, inductive methods are used. Typical questions are open ended without a hypothesis. They invite subjects to contribute to the answers to questions such as "what was your experience when you had acupuncture treatment for your cLBP?" Their answers to such questions are then analyzed. Hypotheses can be generated from qualitative studies. Qualitative research was originally used by sociologists, anthropologists and educators to study people in their "natural environment", in contrast to an "experimental environment" as in quantitative research. It focuses on an individual's understanding of his/her experience and how he or she views about what is happening and the treatment as a whole. Common methods used in qualitative research are interviews, focus groups, questionnaires with open-ended questions, diaries, and reflections. Over the last 20 years, qualitative research has been increasingly used in medical and health research, as the concept of medicine shifts from a biomedical model to a bio-social-medical model (especially in the context of chronic pain). Such research has brought about a wealth of knowledge pertaining to diseases and suffering, and has made a great impact on how medicine is taught and practiced today [5].

We shall present the different types of trial strategies employed to examine the role of acupuncture in contemporary clinical practice, using cLBP as a clinical example. cLBP is a common and disabling disorder, and is the leading cause for visits to licensed acupuncturists [6]. It represents a great financial burden in the form of direct costs, resulting from loss of work and medical expenses, as well as indirect costs [7, 8]. We will also discuss some of the problems and controversies encountered with the current trial strategies, and offer some suggestions for improving clinical acupuncture research.

Efficacy Research

Efficacy refers to the extent to which a specific intervention is beneficial under ideal conditions [9]. A randomized controlled trial (RCT) is considered to be the 'gold standard' methodology for evaluating the efficacy of an intervention. It concentrates primarily on the causal effects of a treatment, e.g., by comparing an intervention with a placebo. While such an approach is typically straightforward in a study of medications, there are a number of issues that make it more challenging to apply to a complex intervention like acupuncture. As such studies seek to isolate the specific effects of acupuncture, the efficacy of acupuncture as compared with some form of sham/placebo acupuncture is frequently used. The questions to be discussed are what constitutes a credible acupuncture treatment and sham/placebo control for acupuncture, and what is the magnitude of the non-specific effects of the sham/placebo controls?

Efficacy Research on Chronic Low Back Pain

A number of RCTs have evaluated the efficacy of acupuncture (verum/real acupuncture compared to sham/placebo acupuncture) for cLBP. A recent metaanalysis[10], which involved a total of 6,359 patients, showed that verum acupuncture treatments were no more effective than sham acupuncture treatments. There was, nevertheless, evidence that both verum acupuncture and sham acupuncture were more effective than no treatment, and that acupuncture can be considered a useful supplement to other forms of conventional therapy for cLBP. These conclusions were supported by a subsequent metaanalysis from the Cochrane Back Review Group [11]. Furthermore, a recent well-designed RCT, which was not included in the above mentioned metaanalyses, also replicated these findings [12].

The evidence thus far has shown that trials comparing verum acupuncture with a sham/placebo acupuncture intervention often report little or no difference between them. The reasons for this could be as follow:

1. Beneficial effects of acupuncture are due to placebo effects and reporting bias [13].
2. Sham/placebo acupuncture interventions are physiologically active [14, 15].
3. Sham/placebo acupuncture interventions might be associated with potent nonspecific or placebo effects [16–18].

If points 2 and 3 can be shown to be correct, it will be difficult to demonstrate a specific effect between verum and sham/placebo acupuncture (see the following text).

Placebo and Placebo Effects

A placebo, as used in RCT, is usually an inactive substance or procedure used as a control in an experiment. The placebo can be any clinical intervention including words, gestures, pills, devices, and surgery [19]. Most CAM researchers prefer the term 'sham', rather than 'placebo', because sham applies better to research on therapies involving devices, surgery, and physical manipulation [20]. The shams designed to serve merely as control conditions may actually produce an effect on subjective or biomarker outcomes. These indirect effects of biologically inert substances or inactive procedures fall under the umbrella term "placebo effects." The placebo effect is a psychobiological phenomenon that can be attributed to different mechanisms, including expectation of clinical improvement and Pavlovian conditioning [21]. Many of the neurobiological mechanisms underlying this complex phenomenon have been studied in the field of pain and analgesia [22].

Placebo effects do not include methodological factors resulting in improvements unrelated to an active alteration of outcome measures, e.g., natural history, regression to the mean [23], Hawthorne effect [24]—a change in outcome measures solely due to being in a clinical study, such as signing a consent form and having some outcome assessments measured, or poor experimental designs, such as subject biases or the purported inert control condition not being inert [25]. The confounding effect of the natural evolution of disease can be solved by including an untreated control group, and proper randomization should take care of the rest. Unlike in pharmaceutical research, however, there is no assumption that the control procedure (sham acupuncture) used in acupuncture studies is inert [14, 15].

Is Every Placebo the Same?

It is generally acknowledged that placebo effect is an important component of any therapy, with treatment effects that appear to be widespread and highly variable. Invasive techniques such as surgery are known to be associated with enhanced placebo effects [26, 27]. Kaptchuk et al [28] reviewed the literature on whether medical devices have enhanced placebo effects and concluded that parenteral placebo is more effective than oral placebo. Furthermore, Kaptchuk and colleagues [29] demonstrated in a separate clinical study that a validated sham acupuncture device (Streitberger needle [30]) has a greater placebo effect on subjective outcomes than oral placebo pills. Their result also showed that the placebo analgesia effect exists beyond the natural evolution of disease, and is detectable over time. This finding is relevant in an acupuncture efficacy trial for chronic pain, as the patients will usually undergo multiple sessions of acupuncture over 1–2 month period, with the outcome measures recorded 3 months to a year after the intervention. A recent Cochrane review [31] on placebo interventions for all kinds of conditions found that 'physical placebos' (which included sham acupuncture) were associated with larger effects over the no-treatment control groups than the 'pharmacological placebos.' Linde et al. [32] reanalyzed the data from this review to investigate whether effects associated with sham acupuncture differed from those of other 'physical placebos'. They separated the trials in which the physical placebo was sham acupuncture from those which used other physical placebos. Their results suggest that sham acupuncture interventions might be associated with larger effects than pharmacological and other physical placebos. However, there is no evidence to suggest that sham acupuncture interventions involving skin penetration are associated with larger non-specific effects than those which do not [18, 33]. The evidence thus far suggests that sham acupuncture control (invasive/non-invasive) is associated with an enhanced placebo effect compared to other physical and pharmacological placebos.

How Large Are the Non-specific Effects (Including Placebo Effect) of Acupuncture?

Linde et al. [18] performed a systematic review of acupuncture trials in any condition, including both sham and no-treatment groups, with a primary aim of investigating the extent of the non-specific effects of acupuncture (difference between sham

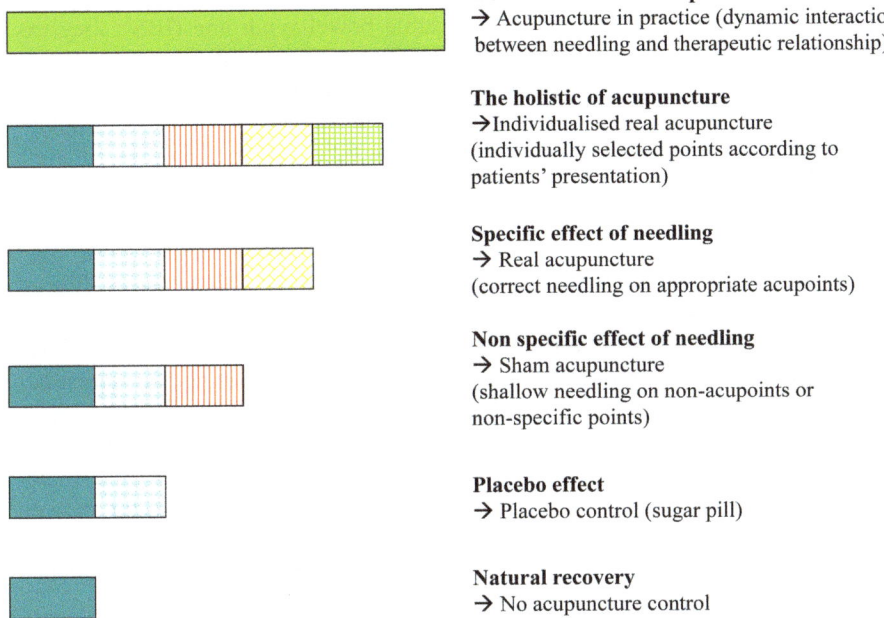

Fig. 7.1 Schematic diagram illustrating the different components of an acupuncture intervention and their contribution to the whole therapeutic effect

acupuncture vs. no acupuncture). Their secondary aim was to investigate factors (such as type of sham intervention, condition, study quality, or intensity of cointerventions) that might influence the extent of such non-specific effects, and to quantify the specific and total effects of acupuncture in the included trials. They concluded that sham acupuncture interventions are often associated with moderate to significant non-specific effects, which could make it difficult to detect additional small specific effects when comparing verum acupuncture with sham acupuncture (Fig. 7.1).

Other factors that contribute to an enhanced placebo effect (and hence, enhanced non-specific effect) of sham acupuncture include the patient's expectations and experience during the treatment. Kalauokalani and colleagues [34] conducted a randomized trial on 135 patients with cLBP who received acupuncture or massage. Before randomization, study participants were asked to describe their expectations regarding the helpfulness of each treatment on a scale of 0 to 10. Their results showed that improved function was observed for 86 % of the participants with higher expectations for the treatment they received, as compared to 68 % of those with lower expectations (P=0.01). Furthermore, patients who expected greater benefit from massage than from acupuncture were more likely to experience better outcomes with massage than with acupuncture, and vice versa (P=0.03). This suggests that patient expectations may influence clinical outcome independently of the treatment itself.

Kaptchuk and colleagues [35] undertook a dismantling approach to examine the placebo effects. In 262 adults with irritable bowel syndrome (IBS), they examined the effects of placebo acupuncture in circumstances involving observation only (evaluating a "Hawthorne effect"), sham acupuncture alone, and an enriched relationship with the treating doctor along with the sham procedure. The doctor–patient interaction in the 'augmented' group involved questions about the patient's symptoms and beliefs about them, a "warm, friendly manner," empathy, communication of confidence, and positive expectations. In contrast, the practitioners in the sham acupuncture only group explained that this was "a scientific study" and that they had been instructed not to talk about it with patients. The results showed that at three weeks, scores on the global improvement scale were 3.8 (SD 1.0) v 4.3 (SD 1.4) v 5.0 (SD 1.3) for waiting list versus "limited" versus "augmented," respectively ($P<0.001$ for trend). The proportion of patients reporting adequate relief showed a similar pattern: 28% on waiting list, 44% in limited group, and 62% in augmented group ($P<0.001$ for trend). This suggests that non-specific effects can produce statistically and clinically significant outcomes and the patient–practitioner relationship is the most robust component. The available evidence so far showed that sham acupuncture is associated with enhanced non-specific effects (including placebo effect), and this enhanced effect can be further reinforced by the patient's expectation, and by the patient–practitioner relationship.

Sham Acupuncture Interventions Are Physiologically Active

A variety of different placebo controls have been used in acupuncture clinical trials. Birch [36] has reviewed the literature and explored 10 research models for conducting sham-controlled acupuncture trials, and discussed the merit and demerit of each in terms of matching the non-specific effects associate with the treatment. Four main types of sham acupuncture were commonly used, based on needling (with/without skin penetration) and point selection (therapeutic point indicated for the condition, acupuncture point not indicated for the condition, and 'non-acupuncture point'/'sham point'):

(1) Skin penetrating: (a) Insertion or superficial insertion at true acupuncture points without further stimulation (e.g., to obtain De Qi feeling). It was felt that this form of sham control carried therapeutic effect and should be avoided. (b) Insertion or superficial insertion at non-acupuncture points with minimal stimulation. This is the most popular form of control used, however, needles inserted into non-acupuncture points and/or superficially used as sham control may not necessarily be inert and may have both specific and non-specific effects [14]. In addition, it remains uncertain as to what constitutes a valid non-acupuncture point/sham point, e.g., true points unrelated to the condition being treated or points located a short distance away from the true points (but located on an area with no known meridian)

(2) Non-skin penetrating: (a) Non-insertion at non-acupuncture points. (b) Non-insertion at true acupuncture points. Non-skin penetrating devices include the blunt

end of a cocktail stick, the needle's guide tube, a tooth pick, and retractable needles (the needle has a blunt tip and retracts into a hollow shaft handle) [30, 37].

Non-insertion devices were introduced to avoid skin penetration and minimize any physiological effects associated with needling. However, evidence so far suggests that both invasive and non-invasive devices can produce the same degree of non-specific effect during acupuncture trials (i.e., non-insertion devices are not physiologically inert) [18, 33]. Historically and clinically, acupuncture intervention has been carried out with non-invasive techniques [38], and non-insertion devices have been available for many centuries. A recent Cochrane review [39] concluded that touch therapies (including healing touch and Reiki) may have a modest effect on pain relief. Kerr and colleagues noted that there are many important common factors shared between touch healing and sham acupuncture rituals (e.g., touch stimulation, the meaning attached to the touch and the modulation of the patient's own somatosensory attention to touch). They conducted a qualitative study [40] by interviewing a subset of acupuncture-naïve IBS patients involved in a single-blind RCT [35], and asked them to describe their treatment experiences while undergoing a course of sham acupuncture treatment. Their results showed that in 5/6 cases, patients associated the sensations including "warmth" and "tingling" with treatment efficacy. Similar touch sensations were also reported by patients in previous accounts of ritual touch healing. In addition, the patients described these experiences as motivating their belief in the practitioner's ability to tailor treatments to patients' specific conditions.

Strength and Weaknesses of Acupuncture Efficacy Research

The main strength of RCT is to preclude biases such as selection bias (by randomizing patients to groups and by concealing the allocation), observation bias (by blinding doctors and patients), and reporting bias (by blinding outcome assessors and statisticians).

Although RCTs provide essential, high-quality evidence about the benefits and harms of medical interventions, many such trials have limited relevance to clinical practice. The investigations are often structured in ways that fail to address patients' and clinicians' actual questions about a given treatment. Efficacy trials dictate that the investigators enrol a homogeneous patient population (with strict inclusion and exclusion criteria), prescribe a standard treatment for all trial subjects to be strictly followed, and inform neither patients nor study personnel about treatment assignments. Thus, although these trials are conducted in clinical settings, their enrolled populations and treatment approaches do not reflect the complexity and diversity of an actual clinical practice such as acupuncture.

Pharmacologic intervention trials generally involve a specific inhibitor, enhancer, or modifier for a specific known pathway. In contrast, although the neurophysiological mechanisms of acupuncture induced analgesia are well established by research for experimental pain, the exact mechanisms underlying the action of acupuncture in clinical practice for chronic pain conditions remains unclear. Walach [41] warned against the use of the existing RCT model to study complementary and alternative medicine, such as acupuncture, as both the verum and sham acupuncture have been shown to generate large, non-specific effects, which occlude any potential specific effects, likely rendering most of the studies under-powered. The explanation as to why many efficacy trials could not demonstrate a difference between verum and sham acupuncture are that sham controls are physiologically active [14, 15, 40], and are associated with potent non-specific or placebo effects [16–18, 34, 35]. If sham control is not inert, sham-controlled trials of acupuncture can be viewed as comparing one form of treatment against another. Furthermore, there is supporting evidence to show that the endogenous opioid system is activated by acupuncture [42], as well as placebo control [22]. Hence, the possibility of type 2 (false-negative) errors in many acupuncture efficacy trials cannot be ruled out [41, 43].

Effectiveness Research

"Effectiveness" is a "measure of the extent to which an intervention, when deployed in the field in routine circumstances, does what it is intended to do for a specific population" [9]. In other words, "effectiveness" reflects whether a treatment is beneficial under conditions close to routine care and, as such, effectiveness studies are also known as "pragmatic" or "practical" trials. Pragmatic trials (PTs) are designed and conducted to answer important questions facing patients, clinicians, and policymakers. The characteristic features of PTs are that they (1) select clinically relevant alternative interventions to compare, (2) include a diverse population of study participants, (3) recruit participants from heterogeneous practice settings, and (4) collect data on a broad range of health outcomes [44]. PTs compare two or more medical interventions that are directly relevant to clinical care or health care delivery (e.g., acupuncture vs physiotherapy), and strive to assess those interventions' effectiveness in real-world practice. However, since neither providers nor patients were blinded to treatment, an observation bias cannot be ruled out.

Effectiveness Research on Chronic Low Back Pain

PTs have been reported in which the effectiveness of acupuncture was evaluated against standard care, or as an overall effect of an additional acupuncture treatment against standard care alone. In addition, these studies also looked into the issue of cost-effectiveness of acupuncture, based on the quality-adjusted life year's measurement. A pragmatic, two parallel group, RCT involving 230 patients was reported in UK [45]. Patients in the experimental arm were offered the option of referral to the acupuncture service. The control group received usual care from their general practitioner (commonly entailing a mix of physiotherapy, medication, and recommended back exercises). The trial protocol allowed up to 10 individualized acupuncture treatments per patient. The acupuncturists determined the content and number of treatments according to patients' need. The result showed that acupuncture care and usual care were both associated with clinically significant improvement at 12- and 24-month follow-up. However, acupuncture care was significantly more effective in reducing bodily pain than usual care at 24-month follow-up. Additionally, the acupuncture service was found to be more cost-effective at 24th month mark. Although the National Health Service costs were greater in the acupuncture care group than in the usual care group, the additional resource use was less than the cost of the acupuncture treatment itself, suggesting that usual care resource use was offset.

Another study involving more than 11,000 patients was carried out in Germany [46]. Patients with cLBP were allocated to an acupuncture group or a no-acupuncture control group. Patients who did not consent to randomization were included in a non-randomized acupuncture group. All patients were allowed to receive routine medical care in addition to study treatment. The result showed that acupuncture carried out on randomized patients as well as on non-randomized patients, in addition to routine care, resulted in a clinically relevant benefit and was cost-effective among patients with cLBP from primary care practices in Germany.

Weiß et al [47] investigated the effectiveness of adding acupuncture in seventy-four patients with chronic low back pain participating in an inpatient rehabilitation program, and compared them to sixty-nine patients who had no acupuncture; both groups of patients received a standard rehabilitation program according to German guidelines. Responses to SF-36 questionnaires showed that the intervention group reported significantly better physical functioning, general health, vitality, and emotional role. Pain outcomes in the intervention group were superior to those in the control group. Specifically, pain with sitting/standing, pain upon carrying loads of 10 kg or more, and prickling in hands and feet were significantly diminished. In addition, 89% of the patients in the intervention group wanted acupuncture to be integrated into standard inpatient rehabilitation, and 83% would even have paid for the service if necessary.

Similar Dilemma of Efficacy Vs Effectiveness Research Involving Invasive Technique in Orthodox Medicine and Its Relevance to Acupuncture

Epidural steroid injections (ESI) is the most commonly performed procedure in pain clinics across the United States for spinal pain and radicular symptom [48]. Two recent systematic reviews of RCTs have failed to show that ESI is more effective than placebo or other treatments for patients with sub-acute LBP, cLBP, or sciatica [49, 50]. These results led Cohen to conclude that it is unlikely that any future trial will provide a definitive answer regarding the efficacy of ESI [51]. Whereas other authors reported favorable outcome following ESI in reviews of effectiveness studies, have commented that it is not realistic to conduct placebo-controlled neural blockade, citing issues of ethics, feasibility, and cost pose challenges of a placebo group; they further suggest that pragmatic studies are considered more appropriate to study neural blockade, rather than explanatory trials [52, 53].

Vertebroplasty (vertebral augmentation)—an invasive procedure which involves injecting liquid cement through a needle into the vertebral body, where it hardens and is thought to restore stability—has been widely used to treat painful, osteoporotic vertebral compression fractures [54]. Two recent RCTs conducted by two independent groups, using sham surgery as control (efficacy trials), have found no beneficial effect. They determined that vertebroplasty is a placebo effect [55, 56]. However, RCTs comparing vertebral augmentation with conventional medical therapy (pragmatic trials) showed augmentation to be beneficial [57–59]. Superficially, it seems that efficacy trials involving all physical interventions may share a similar dilemma with acupuncture, although there are fundamental differences between acupuncture and physical interventions derived from Western medical science (e.g., ESI and vertebroplasty). Traditional acupuncture, as a part of Chinese medicine, is a form of holistic medicine, which addresses not only pain symptoms but also takes care of the root cause identified by Chinese medicine diagnosis. In the following section, we will further explain the components of traditional acupuncture which collectively contribute to the larger therapeutic effect, and its relevance to clinical trials of acupuncture for cLBP.

Acupuncture and Its Effects on cLBP

If one is to apply the same RCT methodology for assessing efficacy and safety for new drugs to assessing acupuncture intervention, the net result of the acupuncture treatment observation may yield a combination of specific and non-specific effects. While the specific effect of a new drug is usually well characterized before it is tested on patients, the exact mechanisms underlying the action of acupuncture in clinical practice for chronic pain conditions is still unclear. However, many recent RCTs continue their emphases on establishing whether there is a specific effect from acupuncture by comparing verum acupuncture with sham acupuncture. This approach assumes that the specific effects of acupuncture are due entirely to needling certain points or to applying certain treatment techniques, without a clear understanding of the complexity of the intervention as practiced in real life (beyond just needling).

Components of Acupuncture Intervention and Their Contribution to the Whole Effect of Acupuncture

A good understanding of what factors contribute to the therapeutic effect of acupuncture is a prerequisite to designing an acupuncture trial, and choosing an appropriate control. For example, the pain relief a patient with cLBP experienced

Table 7.1 Effects of different components of acupuncture intervention for cLBP

Components	Examples
Natural recovery	Fluctuation of chronic low back pain; self-limited nature of acute low back pain
Placebo effect	The perception of being examined and treated brings healing effects
Non-specific effect of needling	Effects induced by needle insertion
Specific effect of needling	Effects from proper needling of points that are shown to be effective for low back pain, e.g., BL23, BL25, BL40
The holistic effect	Effects from needling points that address the Chinese medicine diagnosis or pain or tenderness in other areas and non-pain symptoms related to low back pain. For instance, GB20 is used for neck pain and Anmian for insomnia
Whole system	The total effect is larger than the sum of the effect from each component. This could be due to the interaction between the therapeutic relationship, ongoing diagnosis, needling and outcome of the treatment

following acupuncture could be due to either the whole effect or a combination of the effects from a number of components. These include individualized treatment, specific effects, non-specific and placebo effects, and natural recovery (Fig. 7.1). Examples of the effect of each component are provided in Table 7.1. CLPB often fluctuates, whereas acute LBP is typically self-limited, and both are examples of natural recovery. The specific effects could come from needling, with individual techniques at acupuncture points shown to be effective for relieving back pain, such as BL23, BL25 and BL40. Needle insertion itself would also elicit a non-specific analgesic effect, due to physiological responses to the physical stimulation of needles.

Furthermore, the individualized acupuncture treatment protocol is considered to reflect the holistic nature of traditional acupuncture. For example, cLBP that worsens at the end of the day and is accompanied by fatigue, frequent urination, and shallow sleep differs from cLBP that worsens in the morning, is accompanied with neck and shoulder pain, and is relieved by movement and gentle exercise and warmth. The former presentation is diagnosed as Kidney Qi Deficiency and additional acupuncture points to enhance Kidney Qi, the general bodily Qi, and to improve sleep will be used (e.g., GV2, GV4, BL20, and Anmian). The latter is a typical presentation of Cold Dampness, so additional acupuncture points targeted to alleviate dampness (e.g., BL28 and SP9) and neck pain (e.g., GB20 and SI11) will be used. In addition, moxibustion is indicated to remove coldness from the body. In keeping with the holistic nature of acupuncture, other bodily pains that may or may not be directly linked to low back pain are also treated. Traditional acupuncturists acknowledge body status changes after acupuncture, so reassessing the patient's condition at each session and addressing untreated or emerging problems is an essential part of treatment.

Paterson and Britten [60] consider the whole effect of acupuncture to be larger than the sum of its effects from above mentioned components, due to the dynamic process and the connection between the diagnosis, needling, therapeutic relationship, and outcome. They interviewed 23 patients, who received acupuncture for chronic illnesses, and 8 traditional acupuncturists. Patients and acupuncturists both described the treatment as an interconnected process. A positive therapeutic relationship was viewed as the basis for ongoing diagnosis and treatment by the acupuncturists and as a basis for trust and confidence in acupuncturists by the patients. Positive outcomes also reinforced the trust experienced by the patients. The patients felt they were treated holistically and attributed this feeling to the consultation, diagnosis, the therapeutic relationship, in addition to the treatment. Acupuncture, particularly when carried out in accordance with TCM theory and practice, is a multivariate and complex intervention. Hence, it might not be possible to dissect the individual components and to study them individually.

What Constitutes a Credible Treatment and Control?

Assessment of the effect of acupuncture depends on how acupuncture is defined and what the aim of the study is. Table 7.2 lists these aims, and their corresponding treatments and controls, using cLBP as an example. If the aim is to evaluate the effect of acupuncture alone, then a non-acupuncture treatment control is required to control the 'therapeutic' component due to natural recovery. The treatment should reflect the whole effect of acupuncture, as in some pragmatic trials [61]. If the aim is to investigate some component(s) of acupuncture, this should be stated clearly as the objective in the manuscript. In literature, the most common study design for cLBP is to compare verum acupuncture, involving needling a set of predefined acupuncture points, with sham acupuncture, which involves shallow needling or non-invasive needling on non-acupuncture points [12, 62].

This form of design fits in with the definition of acupuncture given by the National Institute of Health in 1998 [3], "*Stimulation, primarily by the use of solid needles, of traditionally and clinically defined points on and beneath the skin, in an organised fashion for the therapeutic and/or preventive purpose*". However, according to the World Health Organization's definition of acupuncture, sham acupuncture in such a design could be a form of real acupuncture [38]. It defines acupuncture as that which "*Involves the act of needle insertion, although there are many other non-invasive techniques for acupuncture point stimulation. Point may be selected according to: traditional medical system, symptoms, point selection based on the scientific relationships of point function, and point prescription*". Sham acupuncture points commonly used are often in the same neural segments as the real acupuncture points. These sham points could be considered to be real acupuncture points, or therapeutic points, selected based on "scientific relationships of point function". For instance, a German acupuncture trial for cLBP used points on the back as the sham points [63]. However, these points are located within the same dermatomes as the real acupuncture points, and can be considered therapeutic points for cLBP (segmental theory) [64].

Table 7.2 A list of the types of acupuncture treatments and controls using cLBP as an example

Aims of the study	Types of treatment (example)	Types of control (example)
The whole effect of acupuncture	Perform acupuncture per daily practice, allowing all or most of the following items: patient–therapist interaction, • consultations, • other forms of treatment related to acupuncture, such as cupping, moxibustion or electroacupuncture, and • ongoing diagnosis and modifications in treatment	Non-acupuncture control (natural recovery)
Effect of individualized treatment	Acupuncture points selection and needling techniques are tailored to each participant in the group; or treatment selected from a set of pre-defined diagnoses	Treatment with pre-defined acupuncture points for all patients in the group
Effect of specific acupuncture points on low back pain	Correct needling on BL23, 25 and BL40	Correct needling on points that do not reduce low back pain: such as some points on the face ST4 and ST3
Effect of proper needling of acupuncture points on low back pain	Correct needling on most acupuncture points that are effective for low back pain	Incorrect or shallow needling or non-invasive stimulation on non-acupuncture points. This is the commonest form of sham acupuncture control

Furthermore, in sham acupuncture controlled trials, any interaction between therapists and patients must be kept to a minimum to remove the potential for "placebo effect." Such a design does not reflect patients' and traditional acupuncturists' views about the clinical practice of acupuncture, in which consultation is considered an integral part of the treatment [60]. Acupuncturists participating in RCT find themselves restrained when treating participants [40]. The experiences of the patients and practitioners who participated in sham acupuncture controlled trials will be discussed in greater detail later in this chapter.

Finally, the acupuncture point selection in many of the reviewed trials is suboptimal. A recent systematic review [65] of acupuncture for pain associated with the spine shows that, while all the trials chose points on the back and legs with empirical evidence for their effect on cLBP, only two trials employed additional acupuncture points that reduce stress and calm the patients. We consider the omission of treating stress and anxiety to be a deviation from the primary principle of treating pain conditions with Chinese medicine, i.e., to calm the mind of the patients.

While some researchers are still interested in studying the effects of individual components of an acupuncture intervention, they must not confuse that with the whole effect of acupuncture. Ideal treatment protocols need to be established before future trials are conducted.

Qualitative Research on Acupuncture

Over the past 20 years, qualitative research has been gradually introduced to acupuncture and Chinese medicine studies. Some researchers explored patients' perceived benefits, and changes in quality of life and behaviors [66]; whereas others imbed qualitative studies in randomized controlled trials to explore participants' views of taking part in sham acupuncture controlled trials [67, 68].

There are very few qualitative studies about acupuncture for pain. To have a broader understanding of the topic, we have included papers focusing on general changes perceived by patients recruited from Chinese medicine clinics and western acupuncture clinics. Over 60 % of patients who seek acupuncture treatment require pain relief [69]. Three themes have emerged from published qualitative studies of acupuncture for pain: (1) patients' perceived changes after acupuncture or Chinese medicine treatments; (2) patients' perceived differences in the two paradigms of Western medical acupuncture and traditional acupuncture; (3) experiences of patients and acupuncturists who have participated in sham-acupuncture controlled and pragmatic trials.

Patients' Perceived Changes

In a large study involving 460 patients, Cassidy [70, 71] found that a majority of them reported reduced physical and mental pain, improved physical and psychological "coping and adaptive ability" as they became more relaxed and experienced an increased sense of wellbeing, and were able to cope with life better. Furthermore, the patients consumed fewer medications, reduced visits to their doctors, and cancelled surgeries. Her findings have been echoed by other studies [69, 72, 73]. Gould and colleagues [72], and Paterson and co-workers [73] also reported behavioral and cognitive changes, such as change in dietary habit, lifestyle, jobs, and relationships. Subjects also changed the way they look at themselves, such as "learning to live with my body." These cognitional changes usually occurred late in the process of treatment, often after about 21 treatment sessions.

Perception of Acupuncture and Its Relevance to Different Paradigms

Cassidy [71] and Paterson [73] both reported that patients considered Chinese medicine, or the traditional style of acupuncture, to be a practice that treats the whole body and involves close patient–practitioner interaction. Paterson [74] interviewed patients who used western medical acupuncture. Patients reported reductions in musculoskeletal pain and medication use, as well as improvements in mental functioning similar to the results obtained from traditional acupuncture. However, they did not feel they were treated as a whole person because only the primary pain areas were treated and not the areas affected by their pains. This study found that patients who were healthier and had a single problem experienced the most benefit from western style of acupuncture.

Patterson's finding is confirmed by Hughes [75], who directly compared the experiences of patients suffering from rheumatoid arthritis who sought treatment from traditional acupuncturists, western acupuncturists, or both at different times. Hughes found that patients treated with acupuncture, regardless of the therapeutic paradigms, reported reduced pain, improved motilities, and increased sense of relaxation. However, patients experienced broader changes after treatments with traditional acupuncture, especially in their feelings of wellbeing and energy level. They also reported that, in addition to needling, the traditional acupuncturists employed other methods of treatment as well, such as lifestyle changes, as opposed to the Western acupuncturists, who focused primarily on the needling component.

Studies of Participants in Clinical Trials

A group of migraine patients who'd participated in a sham acupuncture controlled trial [67] reported reduced occurrence of migraine and an improved sense of wellbeing. However, they also reported "playing their part" as participants. The participants discovered during the trial that the focus was on acupuncture and migraine, but not on other symptoms that might be related to their migraine. Some patients believed that their migraines were related to certain health conditions, and these conditions were neither discussed nor treated. They also felt that they were not treated as a whole person, and the experience differed from their previous treatments in private acupuncture clinics. The similarities between the experience of participants in this study and those of patients treated by western acupuncturists, as mentioned above [74], are striking.

In another acupuncture trial [40], 12 participants with irritable bowel syndrome who'd been allocated to the non-invasive sham control group were interviewed. Over 80 % reported experiencing a "warm" or "tingling" sensation during the sham acupuncture intervention and associated it with therapeutic effects. It is likely that such experiences result in changes in body sensation, quality of life, and social functioning for this group of participants.

It is also interesting to learn about the experiences of the trial acupuncturists. In a sham acupuncture controlled trial applying a set of formulated acupuncture treatment protocols, the acupuncturists felt the patents were not treated as they should have been in clinical practice, as the acupuncturists could not address other health concerns expressed by the patients [67]. In contrast, in a pragmatic trial, where trial acupuncturists could treat patients in the same manner they would in routine practice, the acupuncturists did not express such constrains—with the exception of two practitioners, who found the number of treatments allowed in the trial treatments to be insufficient [76]. In fact, one study changed its design from sham acupuncture controlled to active treatment controlled trial because the trial acupuncturists considered it unethical to provide the sham treatment [77].

Appraisal

Qualitative studies provide a wealth of knowledge about patients' view of their experiences with acupuncture treatment. The inherent weakness of such studies is that they are retrospective. In addition, selection bias is unavoidable, as people who've benefited from the treatment are more likely to respond to calls for interviews or to answer questionnaires [78]. This data opens another window for clinicians, as well as researchers, who engage in quantitative studies. It challenges the legitimacy of utilizing randomized sham acupuncture controlled trials to examine the efficacy of acupuncture, in which the effect of needling at acupuncture points is the focus of the study. The above-mentioned qualitative studies demonstrate that both the acupuncturists practicing traditional acupuncture, and their patients, consider acupuncture intervention to be a holistic therapy, which not only involves a whole body approach to treating illnesses, but also recognized the healing power of touch and the patient–practitioner relationship. It is time for researchers to step out of the circle of efficacy studies, reexamine the concept and practice of acupuncture, and develop better suited research methods.

Current Status of Acupuncture and cLBP

We consider that the differences between efficacy and effectiveness studies reflect the differences in assessing the components of acupuncture or the whole effect of acupuncture. From the evidence presented for cLBP, moderately strong needling at a set of real acupuncture points (real acupuncture), or an individualized selection of acupuncture points, seem to have little or no specific efficacy when compared with shallow needling at non-acupuncture points (sham acupuncture). However, the whole effect of acupuncture has demonstrated significant clinical effectiveness, and is cost-effective as well, when compared with standard care for cLBP.

Acupuncture is recommended for the treatment of cLBP by some policy makers and professional organizations, including the German Federal Committee of Physicians and Health Insurers [79], the National Institute for Health and Clinical Excellence (NICE) [80], and the American College of Physicians and the American Pain Society [81]. In a recent editorial, Li and Kaptchuk [82] expressed that in our cost-conscious environment, especially when other effective and safe clinical options are unavailable, policy makers have put effectiveness above efficacy. This shift may represent a societal shift in which regulatory and insurance bodies, and "patient-centered health care," have begun to outweigh the "evidence-based medicine" of researchers in determining an intervention's legitimacy.

Some Suggestions for Acupuncture Trials

Based on what has been discussed, we put forward the following suggestions for future acupuncture trials for cLBP and other pain conditions:

1. Terminology changes—All previously labeled "efficacy trials" are in fact evaluating components of acupuncture (e.g., needling/points selection). Researchers should consider replacing "efficacy trials" with trials to "assess the needling components", to avoid the confusion between the effects of components and the whole effect of acupuncture. The whole effect can be examined in effectiveness trials.
2. Investigation of the whole effects vs components effects of acupuncture to further understand the dynamic relationship and their contribution to the whole effect.
3. Design trials to develop optimal acupuncture treatment protocols (in different pain conditions) by comparing different point combinations.
4. Standardizing reporting of clinical research on acupuncture—Researchers should follow The Standards for Reporting Interventions in Clinical Trials of Acupuncture (STRICTA) [83]. These guidelines, in the form of a checklist and explanations for use by authors and journal editors, were designed to improve reporting of acupuncture trials, particularly the interventions, thereby facilitating their interpretation and replication. The guidelines have recently been revised, as a result of collaboration between the STRICTA Group, the CONSORT (CONsolidated Standards of Reporting Trials) Group and the Chinese Cochrane Centre. It is intended that the revised STRICTA checklist, in conjunction with both the main CONSORT statement and extension for non-pharmacological treatment, will raise the quality of reporting of clinical trials of acupuncture [84]. The 'dose' of acupuncture treatment is another aspect of reporting that researchers should pay attention to [85].
5. In addition to a comprehensive and rigorous methodological design, appropriate methods of statistical analysis are also necessary [86, 87].

References

1. Burgess G, Williams D. The discovery and development of analgesics: new mechanisms, new modalities. J Clin Invest. 2010;120:3753–9.
2. Han JS, Ho YS. Global trends and performances of acupuncture research. Neurosci Biobehav Rev. 2011;35:680–7.
3. Consensus Conference NIH: Acupuncture. JAMA. 1998; 280:1518–24.
4. Langevin HM, Wayne PM, Macpherson H, et al. Paradoxes in acupuncture research: strategies for moving forward. Evid Based Complement Alternat Med. 2011;2011:1–11.
5. Bourgeault IL, Dingwall R, De Vries R. Introduction. In: Bourgeault IL, Dingwall R, De Vries R, editors. The Sage handbook of qualitative methods in health research. London: Sage; 2010. pp. 1–16.
6. Cherkin DC, Deyo RA, Sherman KJ, et al. Characteristics of visits to licensed acupuncturists, chiropractors, massage therapists, and naturopathic physicians. J Am Board Fam Pract. 2002;15:463–72.

7. Frymoyer JW, Cats-Baril WL. An overview of the incidences and costs of low back pain. Orthop Clin North Am. 1991;22:263–71.
8. Von Korff M, Ormel J, Keefe FJ, Dworkin SF. Grading the severity of chronic pain. Pain. 1992;50:133–49.
9. Last J, Spasoff RA, Harris S. A dictionary of epidemiology. 4th ed. Oxford:Oxford University Press; 2001.
10. Yuan J, Purepong N, Kerr DP, Park J, Bradbury I, McDonough S. Effectiveness of acupuncture for low back pain: a systematic review. Spine. 2008;33:E887–E900.
11. Rubinstein SM, van Middelkoop M, Kuijpers T, et al. A systematic review on the effectiveness of complementary and alternative medicine for chronic non-specific low-back pain. Eur Spine J. 2010;19:1213–28.
12. Cherkin D, Sherman KJ, Avins AL, et al. A randomized trial comparing acupuncture, simulated acupuncture, and usual care for chronic low back pain. Arch Intern Med. 2009;169:858–66.
13. Bausell RB. Snake oil science: the truth about complementary and alternative medicine. Oxford:Oxford University Press; 2007.
14. Birch S. A review and analysis of placebo treatments, placebo effects, and placebo controls in trials of medical procedures when sham is not inert. J Alternat Complement Med. 2006;12:303–10.
15. Lund I, Lundeberg T. Are minimal, superficial or sham acupuncture procedures acceptable as inert placebo controls? Acupunct Med. 2006;24:13–5.
16. Kaptchuk TJ. The placebo effect in alternative medicine: can the performance of a healing ritual have clinical significance? Ann Intern Med. 2002;136:817–25.
17. Liu T, Yu CP. Placebo analgesia, acupuncture and sham surgery. eCAM 2011;943147. doi: 10.1093/ecam/neq030.
18. Linde K, Niemann K, Schneider A, Meissner K. How large are the nonspecific effects of acupuncture? A meta-analysis of randomized controlled trials. BMC Med. 2010;8:75.
19. Chaput de Saintonge DM, Herxheimer A. Harnessing placebo effects in health care. Lancet. 1994;344:995–8.
20. Hammerschlag R, Zwickey H. Evidence-based complementary and alternative medicine: back to basics. J Alternat Complement Med. 2006;12:349–50.
21. Oken BS. Placebo effects: clinical aspects and neurobiology. Brain. 2008;131:2812–23.
22. Benedetti F, Mayberg HS, Wager TD, Stohler CS, Zubieta JK. Neurobiological mechanisms of the placebo effect. J Neurosci. 2005;25:10390–402.
23. McDonald CJ, Mazzuca SA. How much of the placebo 'effect' is really statistical regression? Stat Med. 1983;2:417–27.
24. Bouchet C, Guillemin F, Briancon S. Nonspecific effects in longitudinal studies: impact on quality of life measures. J Clin Epidemiol. 1996;49:15–20.
25. Kienle GS, Kiene H. The powerful placebo effect: fact or fiction? J Clin Epidemiol. 1997;50:1311–8.
26. Cobb LA, Thomas GI, Dillard DH, Merendino KA, Bruce RA. An evaluation of internal mammary artery ligation by a double-blind technic. N Engl J Med. 1959;20:1115–8.
27. Moseley JB, O'Malley K, Petersen NJ, et al. A controlled trial of arthroscopic surgery for osteoarthritis of the knee. N Engl J Med. 2002;347:81–8.
28. Kaptchuk TJ, Goldman P, Stone DA, Stason WB. Do medical devices have enhanced placebo effects? J Clin Epidemiol. 2000;53:786–92.
29. Kaptchuk TJ, Stason WB, Davis RB, et al. Sham device v inert pill: randomised controlled trial of two placebo treatments. BMJ. 2006;332:391–7.
30. Streitberger K, Kleinhenz J. Introducing a placebo needle into acupuncture research. Lancet. 1998;352:364–5.
31. Hrobjartsson A, Gotzsche PC. Placebo interventions for all clinical conditions. Cochrane Database Syst Rev. 2010;CD003974.
32. Linde K, Niemann K, Meissner K. Are sham acupuncture interventions more effective than (other) placebos? A re-analysis of data from the Cochrane review on placebo effects. Forsch Komplementmed. 2010;17:259–64.

33. Madsen MV, Gøtzsche PC, Hrobjartsson A. Acupuncture treatment for pain: systematic review of randomised clinical trials with acupuncture, placebo acupuncture, and no acupuncture groups. BMJ. 2009;338:330–3.
34. Kalauokalani D, Cherkin DC, Sherman KJ, Koepsell TD, Deyo RA. Lessons from a trial of acupuncture and massage for low back pain: patient expectations and treatment effects. Spine. 2001;26:1418–24.
35. Kaptchuk TJ, Kelley JM, Conboy LA, et al. Components of placebo effect: randomised controlled trial in patients with irritable bowel syndrome. BMJ. 2008;336:999–1003.
36. Birch S. Controlling for non-specific effects of acupuncture in clinical trials. Clin Acupunct Orient Med. 2003;4:59–70.
37. Park J, White A, Stevinson C, Ernst E, James M. Validating a new non-penetrating sham acupuncture device: two randomised controlled trials. Acupunct Med. 2002;20:168–74.
38. WHO: Guidelines for clinical research on acupuncture WHO regional publications. Western Pacific. 1995. p. 66.
39. So PS, Jiang Y, Qin Y. Touch therapies for pain relief in adults. Cochrane Database Syst Rev. 2008 Oct 8;(4):CD006535.
40. Kerr CE, Shaw JR, Conboy LA, Kelley JM, Jacobson E, Kaptchuk TJ. Placebo acupuncture as a form of ritual touch healing: a neurophenomenological model. Conscious Cogn. 2011;20:784–91.
41. Walach H. The efficacy paradox in randomized controlled trials of CAM and elsewhere: beware of the placebo trap. J Altern Complement Med. 2001;7:213–8.
42. Han JS. Acupuncture and endorphins. Neurosci Lett. 2004;361:258–61.
43. Wayne PM, Hammerschlag R, Langevin HM, Napadow V, Park JJ, Schnyer RN. Resolving paradoxes in acupuncture research: a roundtable discussion. J Altern Complement Med. 2009;15:1039–44.
44. Tunis SR, Stryer DB, Clancy CM. Practical clinical trials: increasing the value of clinical research for decision making in clinical and health policy. JAMA. 2003;290:1624–32.
45. Thomas KJ, MacPherson H, Ratcliffe J, et al. Longer term clinical and economic benefits of offering acupuncture care to patients with chronic low back pain. Health Technol Assess. 2005;9:iii–iv, ix–x, 1–109.
46. Witt CM, Jena S, Selim D, et al. Pragmatic randomized trial evaluating the clinical and economic effectiveness of acupuncture for chronic low back pain. Am J Epidemiol. 2006;164:487–96.
47. Weiβ J, Quante S, Xue F, Muche R, Reuss-Borst M. Effectiveness and acceptance of acupuncture in patients with chronic low back pain: results of a prospective, randomized, controlled trial. J Altern Complement Med. 2013 June 5. [Epub ahead of print]
48. Manchikanti L, Pampati V, Falco FJ, Hirsch JA. Growth of spinal interventional pain management techniques: Analysis of utilization trends and Medicare expenditures 2000 to 2008. Spine. 2013;38:157–68.
49. Staal JB, de Bie RA, de Vet HC, Hildebrandt J, Nelemans P. Injection therapy for subacute and chronic low back pain: an updated Cochrane review. Spine. 2009;34:49–59.
50. Pinto RZ, Maher CG, Ferreira ML, et al. Epidural corticosteroid injections in the management of sciatica: a systematic review and meta-analysis. Ann Intern Med. 2012;157:865–77.
51. Cohen SP. Epidural steroid injections for low back pain. BMJ. 2011;343:d5310.
52. Benyamin RM, Manchikanti L, Parr AT, et al. The effectiveness of lumbar interlaminar epidural injections in managing chronic low back and lower extremity pain. Pain Physician. 2012;15:E363–404.
53. Manchikanti L, Buenaventura RM, Manchikanti KN, et al. Effectiveness of therapeutic lumbar transforaminal epidural steroid injections in managing lumbar spinal pain. Pain Physician 2012;15:E199–245.
54. Hargunani R, Le Corroller T, Khashoggi K, Murphy KJ, Munk PL. Percutaneous vertebral augmentation: the status of vertebroplasty and current controversies. Semin Musculoskelet Radiol. 2011;15:117–24.
55. Kallmes DF, Comstock BA, Heagerty PJ, et al. A randomized trial of vertebroplasty for osteoporotic spinal fractures. N Engl J Med. 2009;361:569–79.

56. Buchbinder R, Osborne RH, Ebeling PR, et al. A randomized trial of vertebroplasty for painful osteoporotic vertebral fractures. N Engl J Med. 2009;361:557–68.
57. Wardlaw D, Cummings SR, Van Meirhaeghe J, et al. Efficacy and safety of balloon kyphoplasty compared with non-surgical care for vertebral compression fracture (FREE): a randomised controlled trial. Lancet. 2009;373:1016–24.
58. Voormolen MH, Mali WP, Lohle PN, et al. Percutaneous vertebroplasty compared with optimal pain medication treatment: short-term clinical outcome of patients with subacute or chronic painful osteoporotic vertebral compression fractures. The VERTOS study. Am J Neuroradiol. 2007;28:555–60.
59. Klazen CA, Lohle PN, de Vries J, et al. Vertebroplasty versus conservative treatment in acute osteoporotic vertebral compression fractures (Vertos II): an open-label randomised trial. Lancet. 2010;376:1085–92.
60. Paterson C, Britten N. Acupuncture as a complex intervention: a holistic model. J Altern Complement Med. 2004;10:791–801.
61. Thomas KJ, MacPherson H, Thorpe L, et al. Randomised controlled trial of a short course of traditional acupuncture compared with usual care for persistent non-specific low back pain. BMJ. 2006;333:623–9.
62. Brinkhaus B, Witt CM, Jena S, et al. Acupuncture in patients with chronic low back pain: a randomized controlled trial. Arch Intern Med. 2006;166:450–7.
63. Molsberger AF, Streitberger K, Kraemer J, et al. Designing an acupuncture study: II. The nationwide, randomized, controlled German acupuncture trials on low-back pain and gonarthrosis. J Altern Complement Med. 2006;12:733–42.
64. White A. Neurophysiology of acupuncture analgesia. In: Ernst E, White A, editors. Acupuncture: a scientific appraisal. Oxford: Butterworth Heinemann; 1999. pp. 60–92.
65. Lu SC, Zheng Z, Xue CCL. Does acupuncture improve quality of life for patients with pain associated with the spine? A systematic review. eCAM. 2011. doi:10.1155/2011/301767.
66. Paterson C. Seeking the patient's perspective: a qualitative assessment of EuroQol, COOP-WONCA charts and MYMOP. Qual Life Res. 2004;13:871–81.
67. Paterson C, Zheng Z, Xue C, Wang YY. 'Playing their part': the experiences of participants in a randomised sham-controlled acupuncture trial. J Altern Complement Med. 2008;14:199–208.
68. Kaptchuk TJ, Shaw J, Kerr CE, et al. "Maybe I made up the whole thing": placebos and patients' experiences in a randomized controlled trial. Cult Med Psychiatry. 2009;33:382–411.
69. Xing M, Long AF. A retrospective survey of patients at the University of Salford Acupuncture Clinic. Complement Ther Clin Pract. 2006;12:64–71.
70. Cassidy CM. Chinese medicine users in the United States. Part I: Utilization, satisfaction, medical plurality. J Altern Complement Med. 1998;4:17–27.
71. Cassidy CM. Chinese medicine users in the United States. Part II: Preferred aspects of care. J Altern Complement Med. 1998;4:189–202.
72. Gould A, MacPherson H. Patient perspectives on outcomes after treatment with acupuncture. J Altern Complement Med. 2001;7:261–8.
73. Paterson C, Britten N. Acupuncture for people with chronic illness: combining qualitative and quantitative outcome assessment. J Altern Complement Med. 2003;9:671–81.
74. Paterson C. Patients' experiences of Western-style acupuncture: the influence of acupuncture 'dose', self-care strategies and integration. J Health Serv Res Policy. 2007;12 Suppl 1:S1—39–45.
75. Hughes JG. "When I first started going I was going in on my knees, but I came out and I was skipping": exploring rheumatoid arthritis patients' perceptions of receiving treatment with acupuncture. Complement Ther Med. 2009;17:269–73.
76. MacPherson H, Thorpe L, Thomas K. Beyond needling–therapeutic processes in acupuncture care: a qualitative study nested within a low-back pain trial. J Altern Complement Med. 2006;12:873–80.
77. Coan RM, Wong G, Ku SL, et al. The acupuncture treatment of low back pain: a randomized controlled study. American J Chin Med. 1980;13:181–9.

78. Creamer P, Singh BB, Hochberg MC, Berman BM. Are psychosocial factors related to response to acupuncture among patients with knee osteoarthritis? Altern Ther Health Med. 1999;5:72–6.
79. Brinkhaus B, Streng A. Routine reimbursement for acupuncture in Germany for chronic low back pain and osteoarthritis of the knee—a "healthy" decision? Focus Altern Complement Ther. 2006;11:286–8.
80. Savigny P, Watson P, Underwood M, on behalf of the Guideline Development Group. Early management of persistent non-specific low back pain: summary of NICE guidance. BMJ. 2009;338:1441–2.
81. Chou R, Qaseem A, Snow V, et al. Clinical Efficacy Assessment Subcommittee of the American College of Physicians, American College of Physicians, American Pain Society Low Back Pain Guidelines Panel. Diagnosis and treatment of low back pain: a joint clinical practice guideline from the American College of Physicians and the American Pain Society. Ann Intern Med. 2007;147:478–91.
82. Li A, Kaptchuk TJ. The case of acupuncture for chronic low back pain: when efficacy and comparative effectiveness conflict. Spine. 2011;36:181–2.
83. MacPherson H, White A, Cummings M, Jobst K, Rose K, Niemtzow R. Standards for reporting interventions in controlled trials of acupuncture: the STRICTA recommendations. Acupunct Med. 2002;20:22–5.
84. MacPherson H, Altman DG, Hammerschlag R, et al. STRICTA Revision Group. Revised STandards for Reporting Interventions in Clinical Trials of Acupuncture (STRICTA): extending the CONSORT statement. Acupunct Med. 2010;28:83–93.
85. White A, Cummings M, Barlas P, et al. Defining an adequate dose of acupuncture using a neurophysiological approach—a narrative review of the literature. Acupunct Med. 2008;26:111–20.
86. Shuai P, Zhou XH, Lao L, Li X. Issues of design and statistical analysis in controlled clinical acupuncture trials: an analysis of English-language reports from Western journals. Stat Med. 2012;31:606–18.
87. Lao L, Huang Y, Feng C, Berman BM, Tan MT. Evaluating traditional Chinese medicine using modern clinical trial design and statistical methodology: application to a randomized controlled acupuncture trial. Stat Med. 2012;31:619–27.

Chapter 8
Auricular Acupuncture

Yung-Fong Sung

Introduction

There is a rich history behind the search for effective methods of pain relief and disease treatment. Cultures continually seek out and adopt new methods of alleviating physical suffering, from daily aches and pains to major diseases. The most effective methods have withstood the test of time.

History and Theory of Auricular Acupuncture

Auricular acupuncture (ear acupuncture, auricular therapy) is one of many forms of acupuncture. It is a distinctive part of Chinese medicine that has been practiced in China for thousands of years (Chap 1, 2).

Auricular acupuncture is employed in the treatment of pain and certain diseases by placing fine needles in specifically designated "puncture points" on the external ear. It is simple to apply, with minimal side effects, and often achieves good results. It can be an economic alternative form of patient care with broad applications.

The relationship between the ear, internal organs, and the meridians (acupuncture channels) was first reported more than 2,000 years ago in Huangdi Nei Jing (Chinese Cannon of Medicine). It was compiled during the Warring State period from 475 BC to 221 BC [1].

In a chapter entitled "Kou Wen Pien" in the book of Ling Shu (Chinese Cannon of Medicine) the ear is described as a central location where numerous meridians meet.

Yung-Fong Sung (✉)
Professor Emeritus, Emory University, School of Medicine,
Medical director Emeritus, Ambulatory Surgical Centers,
The Emory Clinic, INC. Emory Health Care, Atlanta, Georgia, USA

When there is internal pathology, whether pertaining to a specific organ or within a body system, the auricle can exhibit external changes such as discoloration, tenderness, decreased electrical resistance in the corresponding meridian pathway within the ear, and even mild morphological changes (scarring) over time.

Inversely, one can also use these changes expressed by the auricle to detect internal organic or systemic disease [2], the so-called "Auricular Diagnosis". The development of acupuncture anesthesia was also based on the analgesic effects on internal organs and whole body systems by stimulating the corresponding area of the auricle.

Dr. Paul Nogier [3, 4], a French neurologist, observed this phenomena in a patient with chronic sciatica who also had scars on his ears. The patient was able to relieve his nerve pain by rubbing certain pressure points on his ear. In the 1950s, Dr. Nogier mapped these auricular acupuncture points and the corresponding somatic representation in the body by developing an inverted fetus map of the external ear (Figs. 8.1, 8.2), similar to the somatosensory homunculus of the brain (Fig. 8.3).

During the 1950s in China, primarily due to shortages of healthcare provisions for the Chinese population and under developed western medicine, general acupuncture—including wide-scale use of auricular acupuncture therapy—was utilized for the treatment of acute and chronic pain as well as treatment for certain diseases (e.g., asthma, hypertension, etc.). Auricular acupuncture was also used as a form of adjuvant therapy in conjunction with narcotics administered for anesthesia. At that time, acupuncture research (particularly auricular therapy research) was highly encouraged by the Chinese government.

Anatomy, Mapping, and Nomenclature of Auricular Points

The ear is mostly composed of cartilage and connective tissue with a minimal amount of adipose tissue, but is supplied with numerous nerves near the skin surface [5]. It is thus often more painful to have needles inserted into auricular points in the ear than into the body.

The ear contains many parts: the helix, apex, helices (tubercle, cauda, crus, and notch), antihelix (including the principle, superior, and inferior parts), triangular fossa, scapha, tragus, supratragus notch, antitragus, intertragus notch, concha, cymba concha, cavum concha, orifice of the external auditory meatus, and ear lobe (Fig. 8.4).

Unlike body acupuncture points, the auricular points were named according to the corresponding parts of the organ or body system (i.e., lung, heart, stomach, endocrine, etc.) [6].

The auricular points are distributed as an upside-down fetus. The ear lobe is related to the head and face region, upper extremities are in the scapha region, the lower extremities are in the superior antihelix crus region, and the internal organs are located in the cavum and cymba concha areas (Figs. 8.5, 8.6a, b).

8 Auricular Acupuncture

Fig. 8.1 Fetus map in the shape of right ear

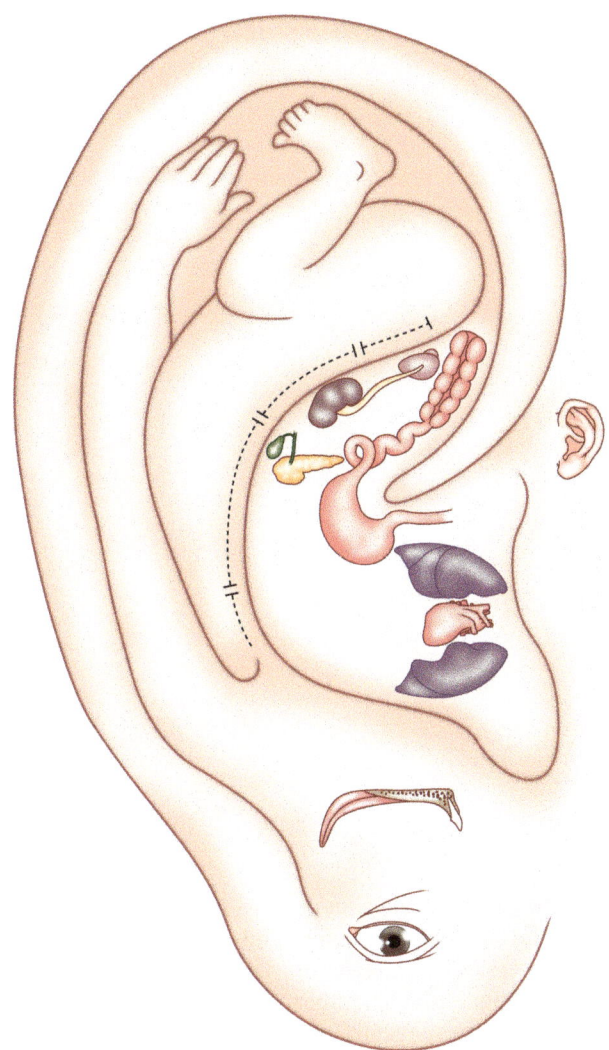

Methods of Auricular Acupuncture

Standard needle: As mentioned previously, needling the ear is more painful than needling the body, even when using the same kind of acupuncture needle. Needles are left in the auricle for 15–30 min to achieve positive results. Overall response is often more effective when employed in combination with concomitant body acupuncture.

Press needle: These needles can be left in the auricle secured by tape for several days in order to achieve long-lasting effects (Fig. 8.7). Particular attention must be

Fig. 8.2 Rear view of left ear

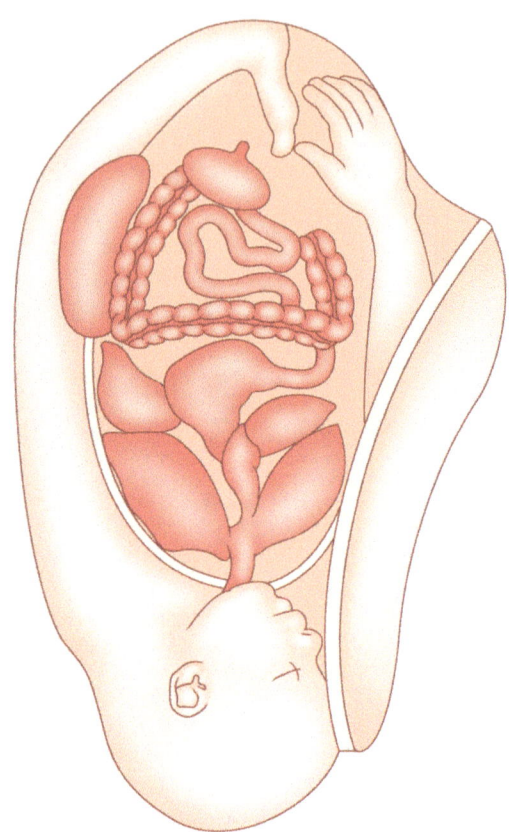

given to cleansing the skin prior to treatment, as there is a higher risk of infection due to the embedding of a foreign body (press needle) over a longer period of time.

Acupressure: Although not as effective as needling, acupressure is a useful tool for self-treatment. A small bead is placed on the skin and secured by tape. It is less invasive and presents minimal risk of infection for long-term treatment.

Other modalities: Electrical stimulation, laser, and ultrasound techniques have also been used effectively on auricular points.

Adverse Effects of Auricular Acupuncture

There are no major adverse effects for auricular acupuncture. Minor effects include minimal hemorrhage or hematoma at the insertion site and increased pain as compared to body acupuncture. Drowsiness and/or dizziness may occur following treatment. The overall incidence of adverse effects is very low [7].

Fig. 8.3 Homunculus of brain

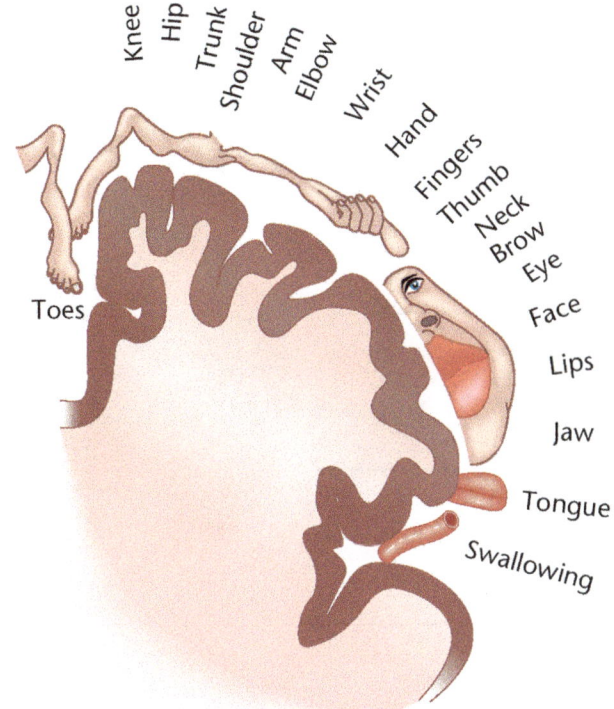

Clinical Applications

Treatment of Pain: When needles are inserted in the appropriate corresponding somatic sites and left for 15–30 min, auricular acupuncture is very effective for the treatment of both acute pain (e.g., decreasing postoperative pain after a tonsillectomy [8]) and chronic pain such as migraine, cluster and sinus headaches, trigeminal neuralgia, and lower back pain [9]. Clinical findings suggest increased effectiveness for pain relief when combined with body acupuncture, particularly in treatment of chronic pain. However, there are some studies that have found *no additional* efficacy of pain relief when using the combination of auricular and body needle acupuncture [10, 11]. Auricular therapy has also long been used in pain clinics in conjunction with other western treatments.

Treatment of anxiety: As per clinical observation, auricular therapy has an increased relaxation effect on the patient in comparison with body therapy. It is not uncommon for individuals to report feeling drowsy after a treatment session. This effect has been useful for the treatment of anxiety, especially in a preoperative setting. Auricular acupuncture is also useful in patients who have a fear of needles, as the patients are not able to see the needles inserted in the ear.

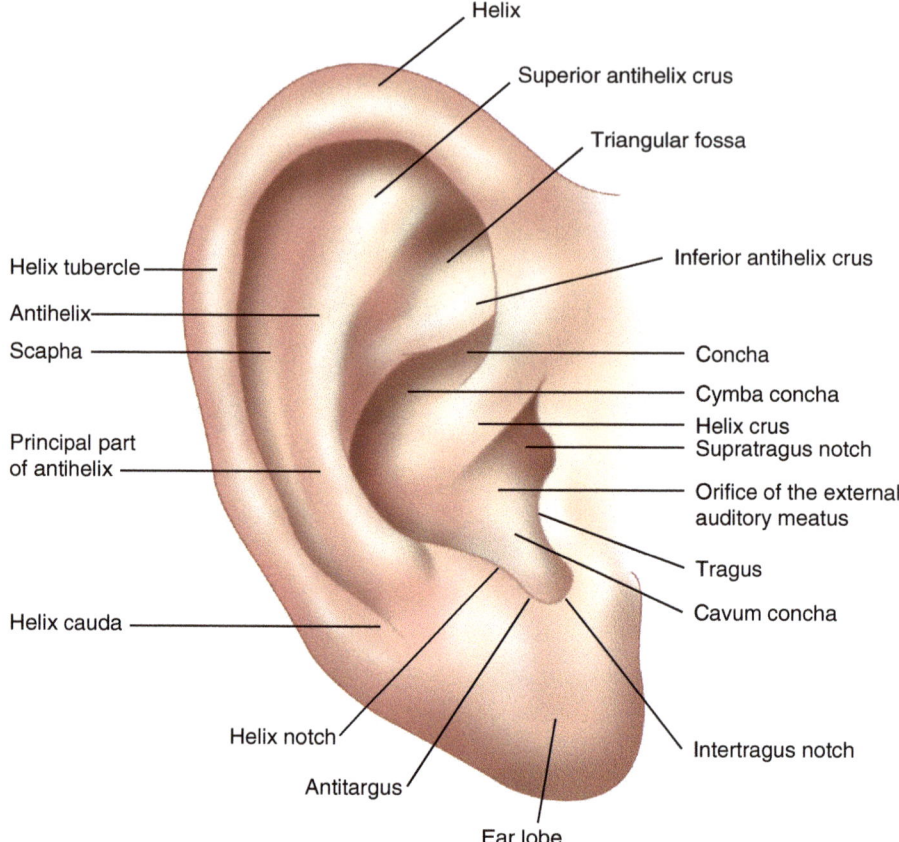

Fig. 8.4 Anatomy of auricular surface

Treatment of hypertension: Although body acupuncture has been known to treat hypertension, there is presently no known study supporting the use of auricular therapy for hypertension.

Treatment of postoperative nausea and vomiting (PONV): Numerous studies have been performed documenting the use of body needle P6 for treatment of PONV. However, auricular acupuncture is not only effective for the treatment of PONV [12], but also patients are often more comfortable during auricular therapy and can use their hands freely during treatment.

Detoxification for drug addiction: There are numerous reports that auricular therapy may assist in treatment for substance abuse of cocaine, particularly in combination with psychotherapy and group sessions [13]. For the treatment of smoking cessation and alcohol dependency, results are still inconclusive [14–16].

Treatment of insomnia: Auricular therapy has been found to be effective for treating insomnia [17].

8 Auricular Acupuncture

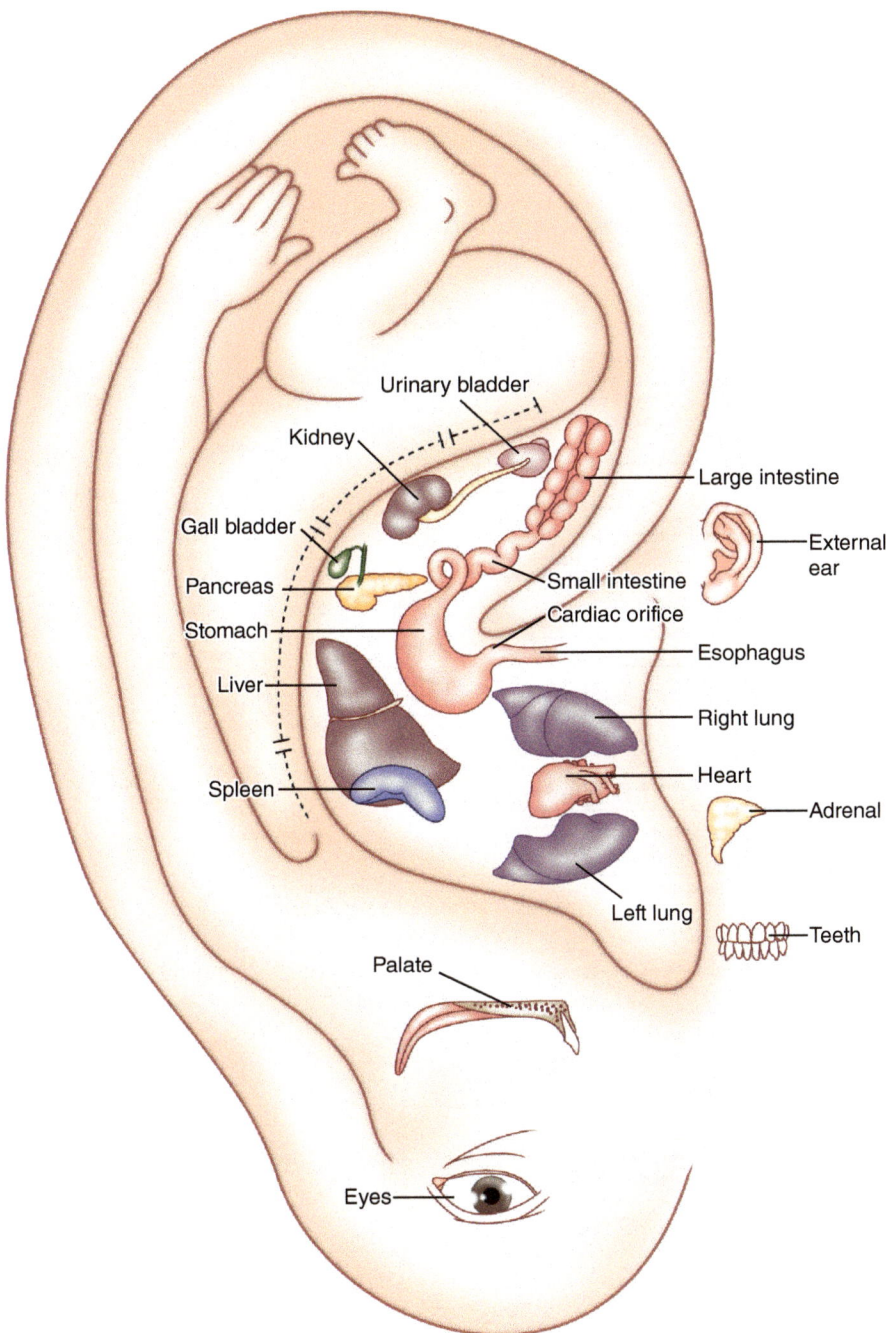

Fig. 8.5 Mapping of the auricular points

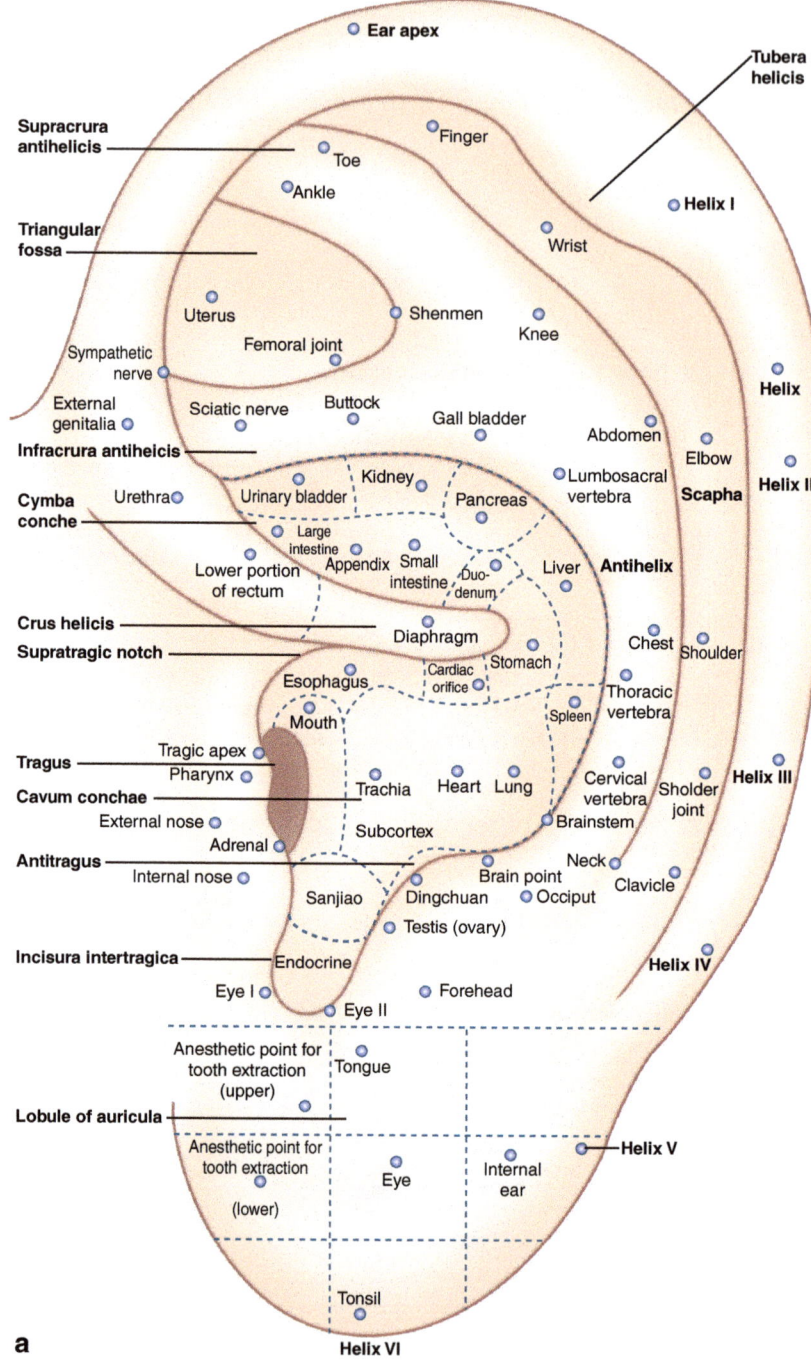

Fig. 8.6 a Detailed corresponding organ and system of the auricular points. **b** Back view of the auricle

8 Auricular Acupuncture

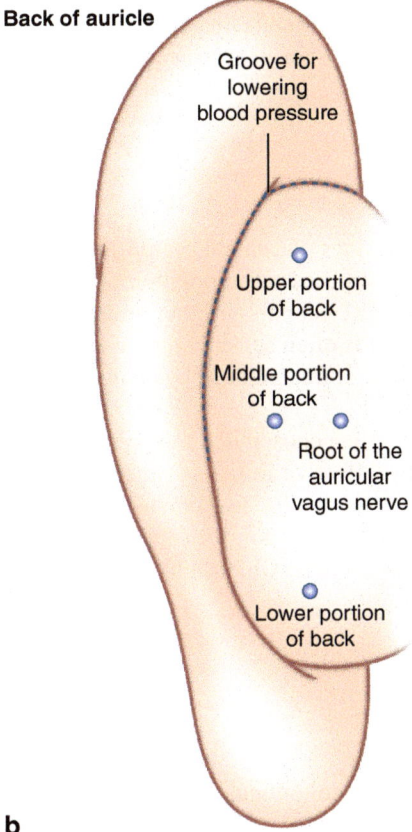

b

Fig. 8.6 (continued)

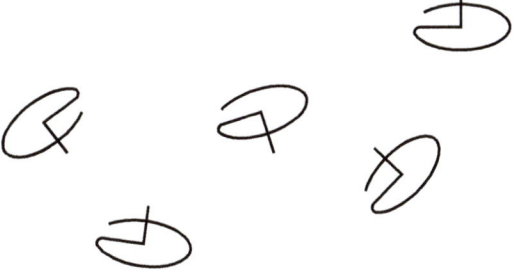

Fig. 8.7 Press needles

Treatment of gynecological problems: There have been several studies demonstrating the effectiveness of body acupuncture for dysmenorrhea, vaginitis, etc. [18, 19]. Auricular acupuncture is effective for hot flashes [20].

Selection of Points

Just as body acupuncture employs placement of multiple needles in specific combinations, auricular therapy often uses a combination of primary somatic points and secondary "assistant" points to treat pain or other problems.

The primary somatic point is often selected on the ear, which corresponds to the organ or system of interest (e.g., treatment of eye pain utilizes the specific somatic point related to the eye).

Other assistant points are then chosen that may not relate to the area of pain but have been clinically proven effective in holistic therapy (i.e., the so-called "shenman" point is known to be effective for sedation as well as pain relief). In the case of eye pain, a third assistant somatic point for the liver is often chosen due to the relationship between the two organs. Chinese medicine theory states that "the eye is the window of the liver".

Conclusion

Auricular therapy is a simple, economical, and effective method for the treatment of various ailments (but especially for pain management) with minimal side effects.

References

1. Veith I. The yellow emperor's classic of internal medicine. 1st ed. Berkley: University of California Press; 1972.
2. Cheing GL-Y, Wan S, Sing KL. The use of auricular examination for screening hepatic disorders. J Acupunct Meridian Stud. 2009;2(1):34–9.
3. Nogier P, Nogier R. The man in the ear. Moulins-les-metz: Maisonneuve; 1985.
4. Nogier R. History of Dr. Paul Nogier's work in auricular medicine. International Consensus Conference on Acupuncture, Auricular Therapy, and Auricular Medicine; 1999.
5. Xinnong C, editor. Chinese acupuncture and moxibustion. Beijing: Foreign Language Press; 1997.
6. Shanghai College of Traditional Medicine: Acupuncture, a comprehensive text. 1994.
7. Ernst G, Strzyz H, Hagmeister H. Incidence of adverse effects during acupuncture therapy—a multicentre survey. Complement Ther Med. 2003;11(2):93–7.
8. Kager H, Likar R, Jabarzadeh H, et al. Electrical punctual stimulation (P-STIM) with ear acupuncture, following tonsillectomy, a randomised, controlled pilot study. Acute Pain. 2009;11(3–4):101–6.

9. Wang SM, DeZinno P, Lin EC, et al. Auricular acupuncture as a treatment for pregnant women who have low back and posterior pelvic pain: a pilot study. Am J Obstet Gynecol. 2009;201(3):271.e1–271.e9.
10. Ceccherelli F, Tortora P, Nassimbeni C, et al. The therapeutic efficacy of somatic acupuncture is not increased by auricular therapy: a randomised, blind control study in cervical myofascial pain. Complement Ther Med. 2006;14(1):47–52.
11. Ahn CB, Lee SJ, Lee JC, et al. A clinical pilot study comparing traditional acupuncture to combined acupuncture for treating headache, trigeminal neuralgia and retro-auricular pain in facial palsy. J Acupunct Meridian Stud. 2011;4(1):29–43.
12. Husang CH, Hsu YW, Chen CC, et al. Effect of auricular acupuncture therapy for the prevention of postoperative nausea and vomiting after gynecological surgery. Taiwan J Obstet Gynecol. 2005;44(3):242–6.
13. Gurevich MI, Duckworth D, Imhoh JE, et al. Is auricular acupuncture beneficial in the inpatient treatment of substance-abusing patients? A pilot study. J Subst Abuse Treat. 1996;13(2): 165–71.
14. Wu TP, Chen FP, Liu JY, et al. A randomised controlled clinical trial of auricular acupuncture in smoking cessation. J Chin Med Assoc. 2007;70(8):331–8.
15. Wang YZ, Chen HH, Yeh ML, at el. Auricular acupressure combined with multimedia instruction in young adults: a quasi-experimental study. Int J Nurs Stud. 2010;47(9):1089–95.
16. Bullock ML, Kiresuk TJ, Sherman RE, et al. A large randomized placebo controlled study of auricular acupuncture for alcohol dependence. J Subst Abuse Treat. 2002;22(2):71–7.
17. Suen LKP, Wong TKS, Leung AWN, et al. The long term effects of auricular therapy using magnetic pearls on elderly with insomnia. Complement Ther Med. 2003;11(2):85–92.
18. Forman A. Acupuncture for the treatment of dysmenorrhea. Am J Acupunct. 1978;(6):139–41.
19. Flaws B. Leukorrhea and vaginitis: their differential diagnosis and treatment. Am J Acupunct. 1986;14(4):305–15.
20. Hammes M, Zhou J, Qu F, et al. Acupuncture and auricular acupressure in relieving menopausal hot flashes of bilaterally overiectomized Chinese women: a randomized controlled trial. Dtsch Z Akupunkt. 2009;52(4):35–6.

Part II
Acupuncture Channels

Chapter 9
Acupuncture Qi Flow and Points Measurement

Yuan-Chi Lin and Cynthia S. Tung

Qi is energy equivalent that runs through the acupuncture points of the body. These acupuncture points are used for gathering, exporting, and converting the Qi flow. Stimulation of the points can facilitate Qi circulation, balance the yin and yang, and promote health in the body. This chapter will discuss these points in relation to one another (meridians) and the methods of measurement employed to locate them on the body.

There are more than 360 identifiable acupuncture points, which are connected along 14 principal meridians. There are 12 paired and two unpaired meridians. The lung, large intestine, stomach, spleen, heart, small intestine, large intestine, kidney, pericardium, triple energizer, gall bladder, and liver are the twelve paired principal meridians. The unpaired meridians are ren and du mai.

The Qi circulates through all 12 paired meridians every 24 h. Therefore, a period of 2 h is the maximum circulation for each individual meridian. This begins with lung meridian at 3:00 a.m. The large intestine, stomach, and spleen meridians follow for the Tai-Yin and Yang-Ming couplets. The Sho-Yin and Tai-Yang couplets begin at 11:00 a.m., which include the heart, small intestine, bladder, and kidney meridians. The Jun-Yin and Sho-Yang couplets begin at 7:00 p.m., with the Qi circulating through the pericardium, triple energizer, gall bladder, and liver meridians (See Fig. 9.1).

Commonly, Yang meridians flow through lateral part of body and Yin meridians run through the medial part of body. The body is also divided into anterior, middle, and posterior. Yang Ming and Tai Yin are in the anterior, Shao Yang and Jun Yin are in the middle, and Tai Yang and Shao Yin are located in the posterior (See Fig. 9.2).

Acupuncture points are commonly located in the depressions, or in the grooves of body. To locate these points, we use proportional body parts as measurement

---

Y.-C. Lin (✉) · C. S. Tung
Medical Acupuncture Service, Department of Anesthesiology, Perioperative and Pain Medicine, Boston Children's Hospital, 300 Longwood Ave., Boston, Massachusetts 02115, USA

Department of Anaesthesia, Harvard Medical School, Boston, Massachusetts, USA
e-mail: yuan-chi.lin@childrens.harvard.edu

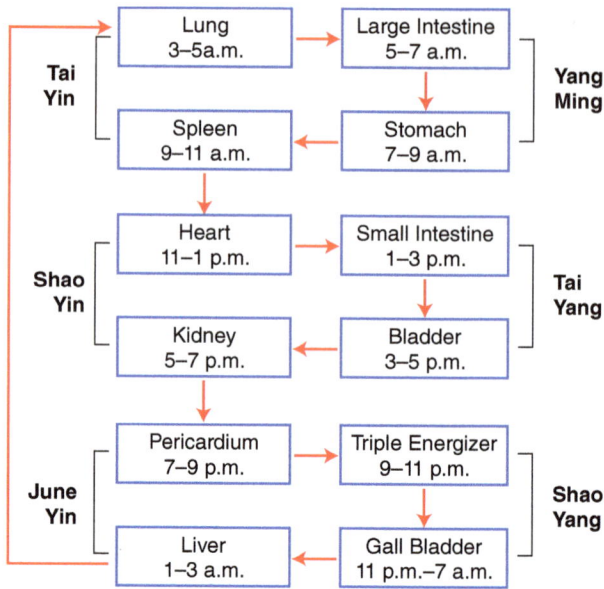

Fig. 9.1 The Qi circulates through all 12 paired meridians every 24 h

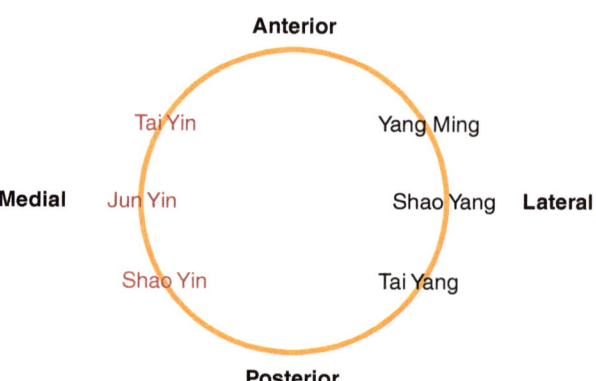

Fig. 9.2 The orientation of Yin and Yang meridians

tools. The distance between the distal interphalangeal joint and proximal interphalangeal (PIP) joint of the middle finger is 1 "tsun" (see Fig. 9.3).

The width of the interphalangeal joint of the thumb is 1 "tsun" (see Fig. 9.4).

If you place the index finger, middle finger, ring finger, and little finger together in a plane, the width of the line across the middle finger PIP joints is 3 "tsun." This is also called 1 "fu" (see Fig. 9.5).

Fig. 9.3 1 "tsun"

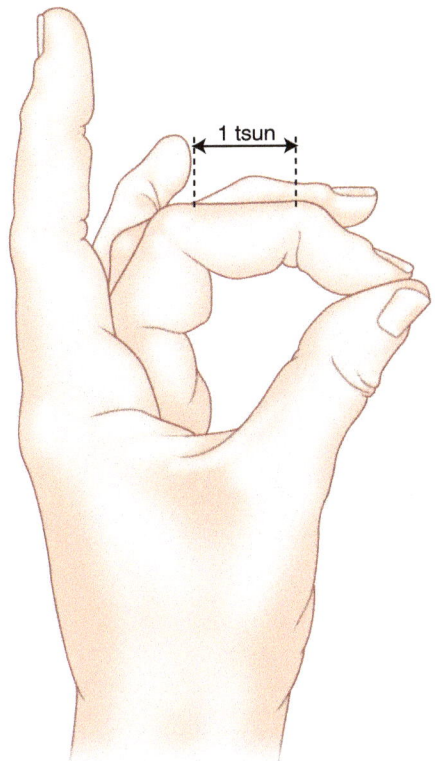

In the head, the distance from the anterior hairline to the middle of the eyebrows is 3 "tsun." The distance from the anterior hairline to the posterior hairline is 12 "tsun." The distance from the posterior hairline to the spinal process of the C7 is 3 "tsun" (see Fig. 9.6) and the distance behind the ear, between the two mastoid processes, is 9 "tsun." (see Fig. 9.7)

In the anterior chest and abdomen, between the sternal notch and xyphoid process, the distance is 9 "tsun." The distance from the xyphoid process to the umbilicus is 8 "tsun", that from the umbilicus to the symphysis pubis is 5 "tsun", and between the two nipples is 8 "tsun."

In the upper arm, the distance from the axial fossa to the transverse crease on the elbow is 9 "tsun" and from the transverse crease over the elbow to the wrist is 12 "tsun."

Fig. 9.4 1 "tsun"

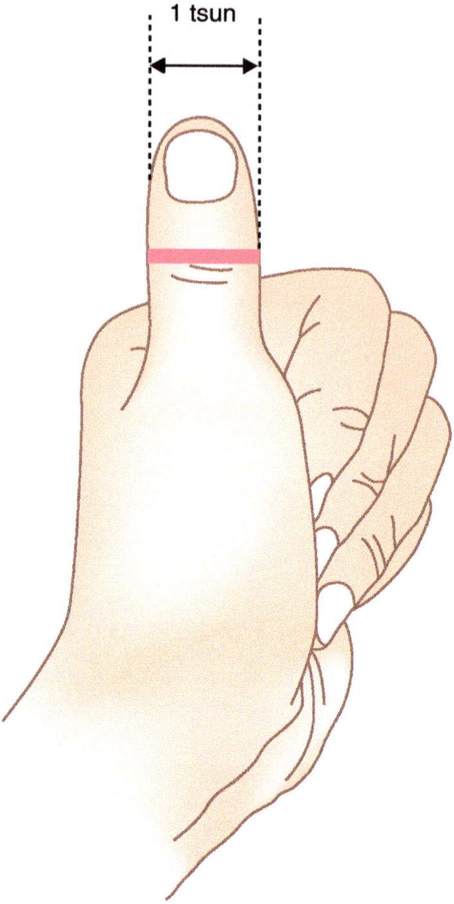

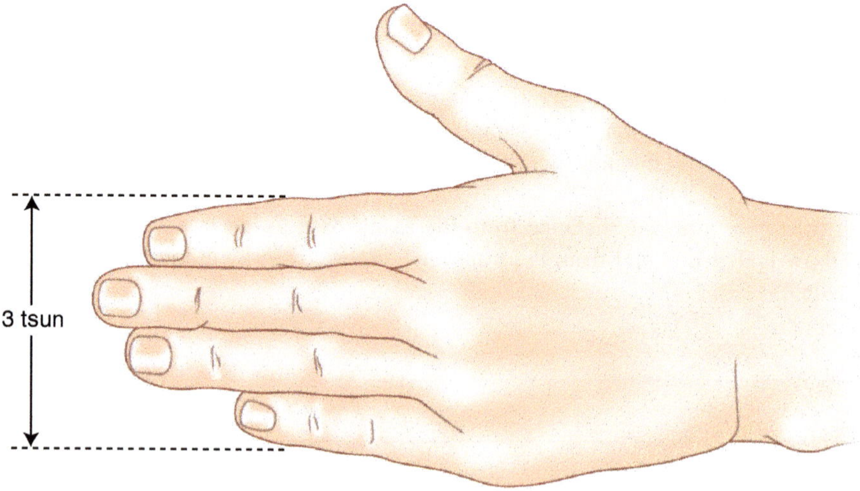

Fig. 9.5 3 "tsun"

Fig. 9.6 Measurement in the head

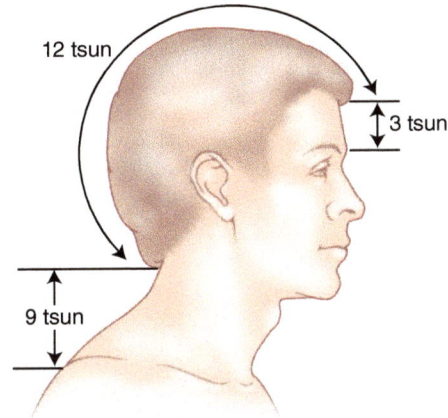

Fig. 9.7 Measurement behind the head is 9 "tsun"

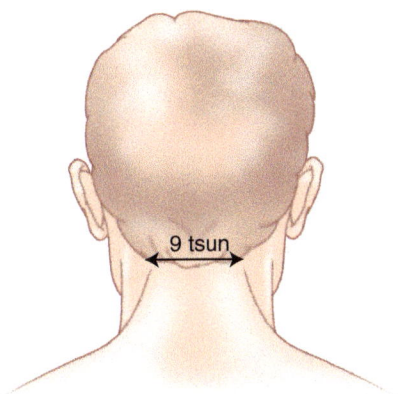

In the lower extremities, the distance from the greater trochanter of the hip to the center of popliteal fossa is 19 "tsun", and from the center of the popliteal fossa of the knee to the lateral malleous is 16 "tsun" (See Fig. 9.8).

Fig. 9.8 Measurement in the anterior chest and abdomen, the upper arm, and the lower extremities

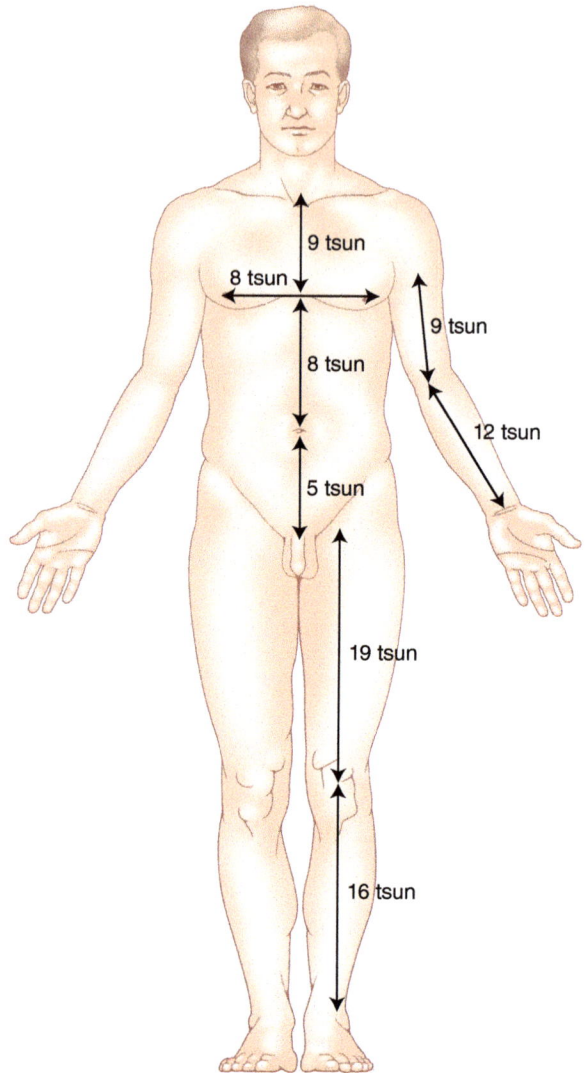

Chapter 10
Hand Tai Yin Lung Meridian 手太陰肺經穴

Yuan-Chi Lin and Rosalie F. Tassone

LU 1 Zhongfu 中府	On the anterior thoracic region, at the same level as the first intercostal space, lateral to the infraclavicular fossa, 6 B-cun lateral to the anterior median line.
LU 2 Yunmen 雲門	On the anterior thoracic region, in the depression of the infraclavicular fossa, medial to the coracoid process of the scapula, 6 B-cun lateral to the anterior median line.
LU 3 Tianfu 天府	On the anterolateral aspect of the arm, just lateral to the border of the biceps brachii muscle, 3 B-cun inferior to the anterior axillary fold.
LU 4 Xiabai 俠白	On the anterolateral aspect of the arm, just lateral to the border of the biceps brachii muscle, 4 B-cun inferior to the anterior axillary fold.
LU 5 Chize 尺澤	On the anterior aspect of the elbow, at the cubital crease, in the depression lateral to the biceps brachii tendon.
LU 6 Kongzui 孔最	On the anterolateral aspect of the forearm, on the line connecting LU 5 with LU 9, 7 B-cun superior to the palmar wrist crease.
LU 7 Lieque 列缺	On the radial aspect of the forearm, between the tendons of the abductor pollicis longus and the extensor pollicis brevis muscles, in the groove for the abductor pollicis longus tendon, 1.5 B-cun superior to the palmar wrist crease.

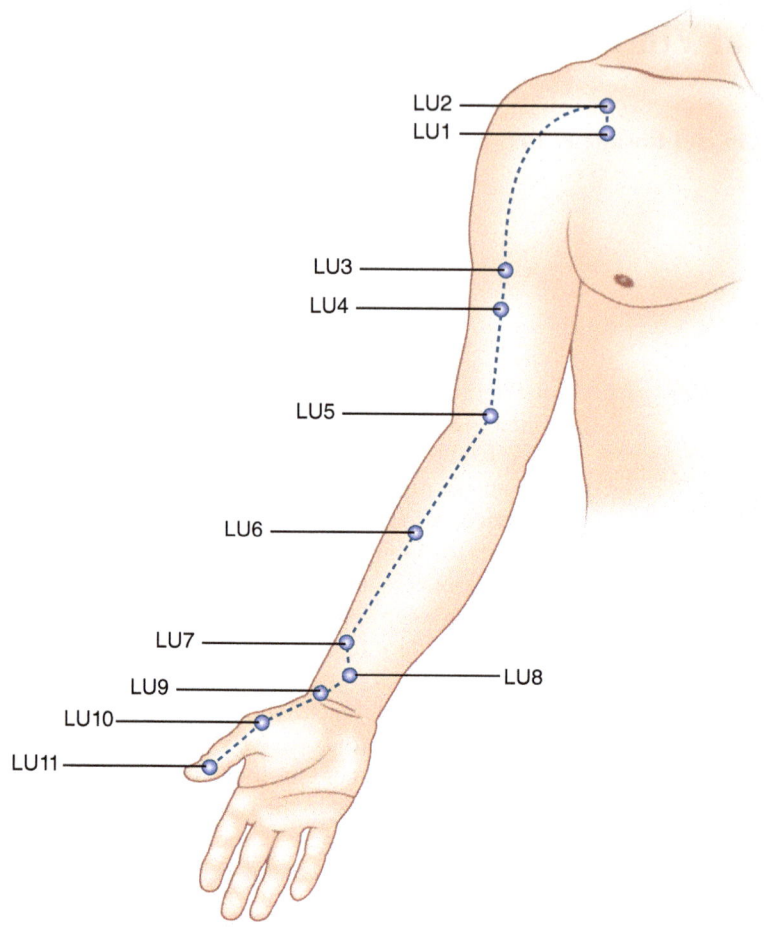

Fig. 10.1 Hand Tai Yin lung meridian

LU 8 Jingqu 經渠	On the anterolateral aspect of the forearm, between the radial styloid process and the radial artery, 1 B-cun superior to the palmar wrist crease.
LU 9 Taiyuan 太淵	On the anterolateral aspect of the wrist, between the radial styloid process and the scaphoid bone, in the depression ulnar to the abductor pollicis longus tendon.
LU 10 Yuji 魚際	On the palm, radial to the midpoint of the first metacarpal bone, at the border between the red and white flesh.
LU 11 Shaoshang 少商	On the radial side of the thumb nail, at the junction of the vertical line of radial nail border and the horizontal line of the base of thumb nail (see Fig. 10.1).

Chapter 11
Hand Yang Ming Large Intestine Meridian
手陽明大腸經穴

Yuan-Chi Lin and Rosalie F. Tassone

LI 1 Shangyang 商陽	On the radial side of index finger nail bed, 0.1 tsun proximal to the corner of nail.
LI 2 Erjian 二間	On the radial side of the index finger, distal to the metaphalangeal joint.
LI 3 Sanjian 三間	On the radial side of the distal part of second metacarpal bone.
LI 4 Hegu 合谷	On the dorsum of the hand, between the first and second metacarpal bones, radial to the midpoint of the second metacarpal bone.
LI 5 Yangxi 陽谿	Over the posterolateral aspect of wrist joint, between the tendons of extensor pollicis longus and extensor pollicis brevis.
LI 6 Pianli 偏歷	On the posterolateral aspect of the forearm, 3 tsun proximal to the LI 5 Yangxi.
LI 7 Wenliu 溫溜	On the radial and dorsal side of forearm, 5 tsun proximal to the dorsal wrist crease Yangxi.
LI 8 Xialian 下廉	On the posterolateral aspect of the forearm, 4 tsun inferior to the Quchi and 3 tsum superior to the Wenliu.
LI 9 Shanglian 上廉	On the posterolateral aspect of the forearm, 3 tsun inferior to the Quchi and 1 tsum superior to the Xialian.
LI 10 Shousanli 手三里	Two tsun distal to the point LI 11 on the line connecting LI 11 and LI 5.

Y.-C. Lin (✉)
Medical Acupuncture Service, Department of Anesthesiology, Perioperative and Pain Medicine,
Boston Children's Hospital, 300 Longwood Ave., Boston, Massachusetts 02115, USA

Department of Anaesthesia, Harvard Medical School, Boston, Massachusetts, USA
e-mail: yuan-chi.lin@childrens.harvard.edu

R. F. Tassone
Department of Anesthesiology, University of Illinois at Chicago,
1740 West Taylor Street, Chicago, Illinois 60612, USA
e-mail: rtassone@uic.edu

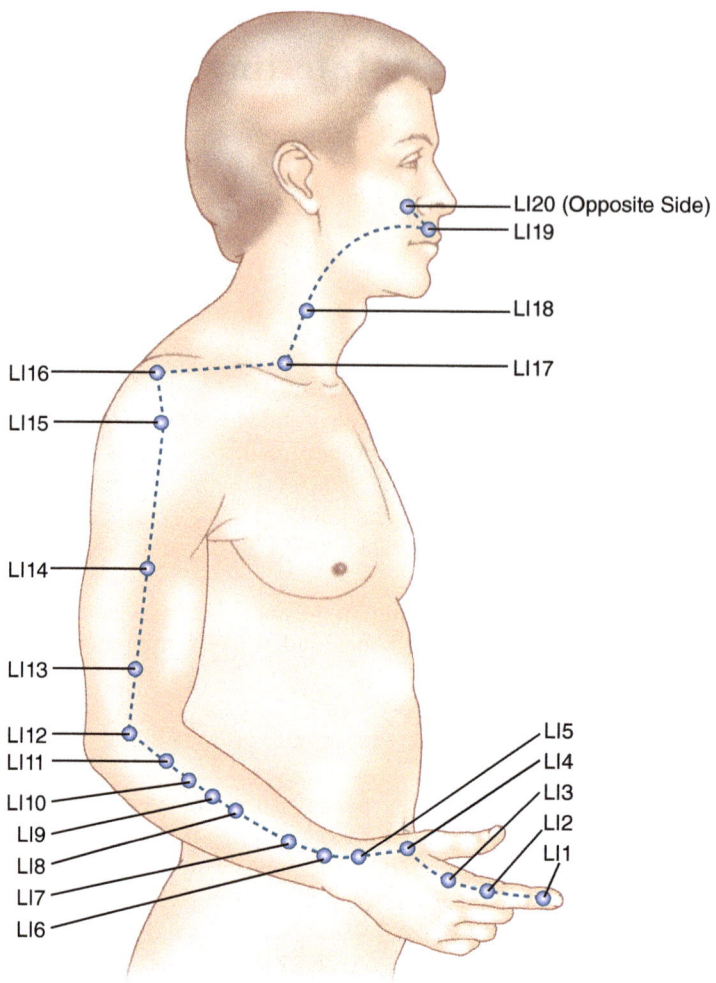

Fig. 11.1 Hand Yang Ming large intestine meridian

LI 11 Quchi 曲池	At the lateral aspect of elbow, at the end of lateral transverse crease.
LI 12 Zhouliao 肘髎	At the lateral aspect of elbow, superior to the lateral epicondyle of the humerus.
LI 13 Shouwuli 手五里	On the lateral aspect of arm, 3 tsun proximal to the elbow crease.
LI 14 Binao 臂臑	On the lateral aspect of arm, 7 tsun proximal to the elbow crease.

11 Hand Yang Ming Large Intestine Meridian 手陽明大腸經穴

LI 15 Jianyu 肩髃	On the anterior depression of shoulder, between the anterior end of lateral border of the acromion and the greater tubercle of the humerus, at the corner of the shoulder.
LI 16 Jugu 巨骨	At the depression between the acromial end of the clavicle and the upper part of the spine of scapula.
LI 17 Tianding 天鼎	On the anterior aspect of neck, at the posterior margin of sternocleidomastoid muscle, at the level of cricoids cartilage.
LI 18 Futu 扶突	On the anterior aspect of neck, at the level of superior level of thyroid cartilages, between the anterior and posterior border sternocleidomastoid muscles.
LI 19 Heliao 口禾髎	On the face, inferior to the lateral margin of nostril at the same level as the midpoint of the philtrum.
LI 20 Yingxiang 迎香	On the face, at the junction of ala nasi and the nasolabial groove (Fig. 11.1).

Chapter 12
Foot Yang Ming Stomach Meridian
足陽明胃經穴

Yuan-Chi Lin and Rosalie F. Tassone

ST 1 Chengqi 承泣	On the depression in the midline of lower eyelid.
ST 2 Sibai 四白	Three tsun below ST 1, in the depression at the infra-orbital foramen.
ST 3 Juliao 巨髎	Directly below the midline of lower eyelid at the level of lower border of the ala of nose.
ST 4 Dicang 地倉	Half tsun lateral to the corner of the mouth.
ST 5 Daying 大迎	Anterior to the angle of mandible, in the depression anterior to the masseter attachment.
ST 6 Jiache 頰車	One-finger breadth anterior and superior to the angle of the mandible.
ST 7 Xiaguan 下關	On the lateral of face, in the depression between midpoint below of the lateral zygomatic arch and mandibular notch.
ST 8 Touwei 頭維	Half tsun within the ideal hairline at the corner of the forehead; 4.5 tsun lateral to the midline.
ST 9 Renyins 人迎	At the anterior margin of the sternocleidomastoid muscle at the level of upper border of thyroid cartilage.
ST 10 Shuitu 水突	At the anterior margin of the sternocleidomastoid muscle at the level of upper border of cricoids cartilage.
ST 11 Qishe 氣舍	Above the clavicle at the depression between sterna head and clavicle head of sternocleidomastoid muscle.
ST 12 Quepen 缺盆	At supraclavicle fossa 4 tsun lateral to the anterior median line of the neck.

Y.-C. Lin (✉)
Medical Acupuncture Service, Department of Anesthesiology, Perioperative and Pain Medicine, Boston Children's Hospital, 300 Longwood Ave., Boston, Massachusetts 02115, USA

Department of Anaesthesia, Harvard Medical School, Boston, Massachusetts, USA
e-mail: yuan-chi.lin@childrens.harvard.edu

R. F. Tassone
Department of Anesthesiology, University of Illinois at Chicago,
1740 West Taylor Street, Chicago, Illinois 60612, USA
e-mail: rtassone@uic.edu

ST 13 Qihu 氣户	At infraclavicle fossa 4 tsun lateral to the anterior median line of the neck.
ST 14 Kufang 庫房	At first intercostals space 4 tsun lateral to the anterior median line of the chest.
ST 15 Wuyi 屋翳	At second intercostals space 4 tsun lateral to the anterior median line of the chest.
ST 16 Yingchuang 膺窗	At third intercostals space 4 tsun lateral to the anterior median line of the chest.
ST 17 Ruzhong 乳中	At the center of the nipple.
ST 18 Rugen 乳根	At fifth intercostals space 4 tsun lateral to the anterior median line of the chest.
ST 19 Burong 不容	On the upper abdomen, 2 tsun lateral to the anterior median line, 6 tsun above the umbilicus.
ST 20 Chengman 承滿	On the upper abdomen, 2 tsun lateral to the anterior median line and 5 tsun above the umbilicus.
ST 21 Liangmen 梁門	On the upper abdomen, 2 tsun lateral to the anterior median line, 4 tsun above the umbilicus.
ST 22 Guanmen 關門	On the upper abdomen, 2 tsun lateral to the anterior median line, 3 tsun above the umbilicus.
ST 23 Taiyi 太乙	On the upper abdomen, 2 tsun lateral to the anterior median line, 2 tsun above the umbilicus.
ST 24 Huaroumen 滑肉門	On the upper abdomen, 2 tsun lateral to the anterior median line, 1 tsun above the umbilicus.
ST 25 Tianshu 天樞	On the upper abdomen, 2 tsun lateral to the umbilicus.
ST 26 Wailing 外陵	On the upper abdomen, 2 tsun lateral to the anterior median line, 1 tsun inferior the umbilicus.
ST 27 Daju 大巨	On the upper abdomen, 2 tsun lateral to the anterior median line, 2 tsun inferior the umbilicus.
ST 28 Shuidao 水道	On the upper abdomen, 2 tsun lateral to the anterior median line, 3 tsun inferior the umbilicus.
ST 29 Guilai 歸來	On the upper abdomen, 2 tsun lateral to the anterior median line, 4 tsun inferior the umbilicus.
ST 30 Qichong 氣衝	On the upper abdomen, 2 tsun lateral to the anterior median line, 5 tsun inferior the umbilicus.
ST 31 Biguan 髀關	On the anterior thigh, below the anterior superior iliac spine, in the depression lateral side of the sartorius muscle.
ST 32 Futu 伏兔	On the anterior thigh, on the line connecting anterior iliac spine and lateral border of patella, 6 tsun proximal to the superior lateral border of patella.
ST 33 Yinshi 陰市	On the anterior thigh, on the line connecting anterior iliac spine and lateral border of patella, 3 tsun proximal to the superior lateral border of patella.
ST 34 Liangqiu 梁丘	Two tsun proximal to the superior lateral corner border of patella.

12 Foot Yang Ming Stomach Meridian 足陽明胃經穴

Fig. 12.1 Foot Yang Ming stomach meridian

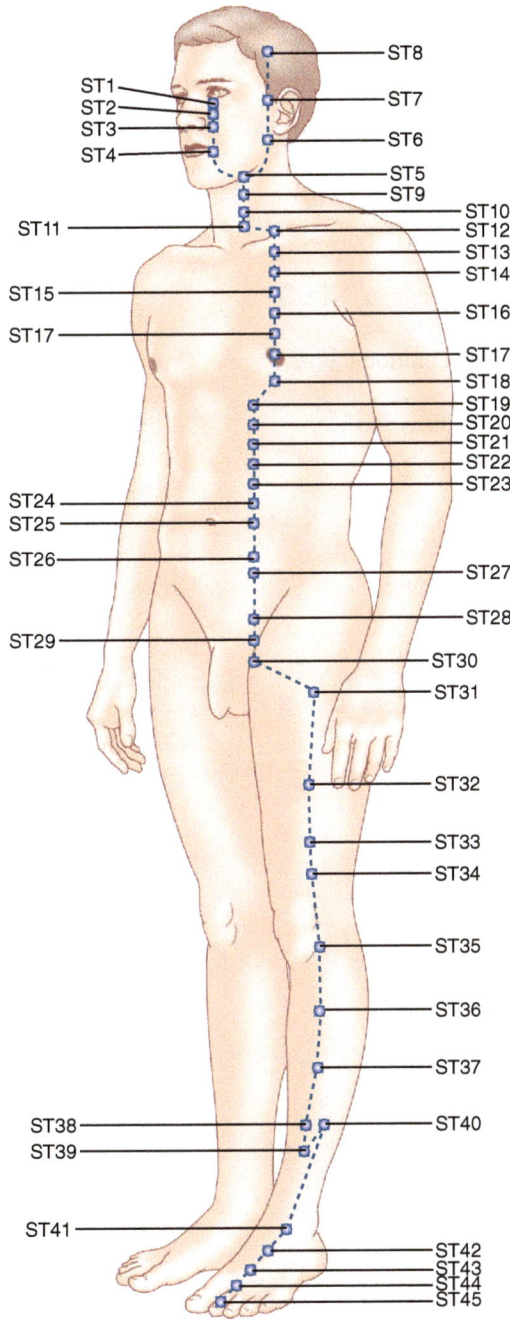

ST 35 Dubi 犢鼻	Over the deep depression inferior and lateral of patella.
ST 36 Zusanli 足三里	Three tsun below the ST 35; 1 tsun lateral to the anterior crest of the tibia.
ST 37 Shangjuxu 上巨虛	Three tsun below the ST 36; 1 tsun lateral to the anterior crest of the tibia.
ST 38 Tiaokou 條口	Two tsun below ST 37; 1 tsun lateral to the anterior crest of the tibia; it locates at the midpoint between ST 35 and ST 41.
ST 39 Xiajuxu 下巨虛	Three tsun below ST 37; 1 tsun lateral to the anterior crest of the tibia.
ST 40 Fenglong 豐隆	One finger width lateral to ST 38; 8 tsun distal to ST 35.
ST 41 Jiexi 解谿	At the junction between the dorsum of foot and leg; between tendons of extensor hallucis longus and extensor digitorum longus.
ST 42 Chongyang 衝陽	On the dorsum of foot, proximal to the base between the second and third metatarsal bones.
ST 43 Xiangu 陷谷	On the dorsum of foot, in the depression distal to the junction of the second and third metatarsal bones.
ST 44 Neiting 内庭	On the dorsum of the foot, at the edge of the interdigital skin between the second and third toe.
ST 45 Lidui 厲兌	On the lateral side of the second toe proximal to the corner of the nail (see Fig. 12.1).

Chapter 13
Foot Tai Yin Spleen Meridian 足太陰脾經穴

Yuan-Chi Lin and Rosalie F. Tassone

SP 1 Yinbai 隱白	On the medial side of big toe, 0.1 tsun posterior to the corner of the medial side of big toe.
SP 2 Dadu 大都	On the medial side of big toe, in the depression distal to the first metatarsophalangeal joint.
SP 3 Taibai 太白	On the medial side of big toe, in the depression proximal to the first metatarsophalangeal joint.
SP 4 Gongsun 公孫	On the medical aspect of foot, anterior inferior border of the proximal end of first metatarsal bone.
SP 5 Shansqiu 商丘	In the depression over the anterior-inferior to the medial malleolus.
SP 6 Sanyinjiao 三陰交	Posterior to the border of tibia, 3 tsun proximal to the medial malleolus.
SP 7 Logu 漏谷	Posterior to the border of tibia, 6 tsun proximal to the medial malleolus.
SP 8 Diji 地機	At the posterior border of tibia, 3 tsun distal to the medial condyle of tibia.
SP 9 Yinlingquan 陰陵泉	At the medial side inferior to the knee, in the depression of lower border of medial condyle.
SP 10 Xuehai 血海	Two tsun proximal to the upper medial border of patella.
SP 11 Jimen 箕門	On the medial side of Sartorius muscle, 6 tsun proximal to the SP 10.
SP 12 Chongmen 衝門	In the groin region, lateral to the femoral artery.

Y.-C. Lin (✉)
Medical Acupuncture Service, Department of Anesthesiology, Perioperative and Pain Medicine, Boston Children's Hospital, 300 Longwood Ave., Boston, Massachusetts 02115, USA

Department of Anaesthesia, Harvard Medical School, Boston, Massachusetts, USA
e-mail: yuan-chi.lin@childrens.harvard.edu

R. F. Tassone
Department of Anesthesiology, University of Illinois at Chicago,
1740 West Taylor Street, Chicago, Illinois 60612, USA,
e-mail: rtassone@uic.edu

Y.-C. Lin, E. S.-Z. Hsu (eds.), *Acupuncture for Pain Management*,
DOI 10.1007/978-1-4614-5275-1_13, © Springer Science+Business Media New York 2014

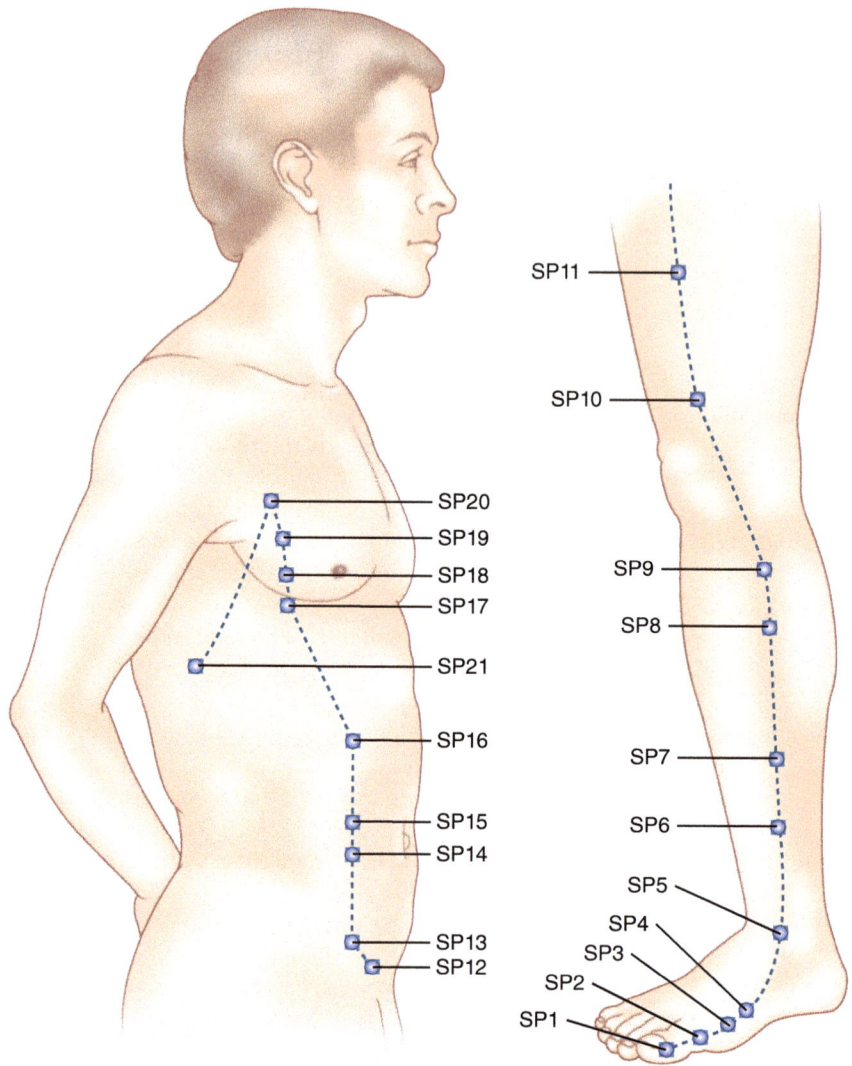

Fig. 13.1 Foot Tai Yin spleen meridian

SP 13 Fushe 府舍	Four tsun lateral to the midline, 0.7 tsun superior to the SP 12.
SP 14 Fujie 腹结	On the low abdomen, 1.3 tsun below the umbilicus and 4 tsun lateral to the anterior median line.
SP 15 Daheng 大横	In the abdomen, 4 tsun lateral to the umbilicus.
SP 16 Fuai 腹哀	On the upper abdomen, 3 tsun above the umbilicus and 4 tsun lateral to the anterior median line.

13 Foot Tai Yin Spleen Meridian 足太陰脾經穴

SP 17 Shidou 食竇	In the anterior thoracic region, at the fifth intercostals space, 6 tsun lateral to the anterior meddle line.
SP 18 Tianxi 天谿	In the anterior thoracic region, at the fourth intercostals space, 6 tsun lateral to the anterior meddle line.
SP 19 Xiongxiang 胸鄉	In the anterior thoracic region, at the third intercostals space, 6 tsun lateral to the anterior meddle line.
SP 20 Zhourong 周榮	In the anterior thoracic region, at the second intercostals space, 6 tsun lateral to the anterior meddle line.
SP 21 Dabao 大包	In the lateral thoracic region, at the sixth intercostals space, in the mid axillary line (see Fig. 13.1).

Chapter 14
The Hand Shao Yin Heart Meridian
手少陰心經穴

Rosalie F. Tassone and Yuan-Chi Lin

HT 1 Jiquan 極泉	In the center of the axilla fossa.
HT 2 Qingling 青靈	On the medial aspect of arm, 3 tsun proximal to the medial end of transverse cubital crease.
HT 3 Shaohai 少海	On the medial aspect of elbow, at the medial end of transverse cubital crease, in the depression anterior to the medial epicondyle.
HT 4 Lingdao 靈道	On the anteromedial aspect of forearm, 1.5 tsun proximal to the palmar wrist crease, between the tendons of flexor digitorum superficialis and flexor carpi ulnaris muscles.
HT 5 Tongli 通里	On the anteromedial aspect of forearm, 1 tsun proximal to the palmar wrist crease, between the tendons of flexor digitorum superficialis and flexor carpi ulnaris muscles.
HT 6 Yinxi 陰郄	On the anteromedial aspect of forearm, 0.5 tsun proximal to the palmar wrist crease, between the tendons of flexor digitorum superficialis and flexor carpi ulnaris muscles.
HT 7 Shenmen 神門	On the anteromedial aspect of forearm and on the palmar wrist crease, radial to the tendon of the flexor carpi ulnaris muscle.

R. F. Tassone (✉)
Department of Anesthesiology, University of Illinois at Chicago,
1740 West Taylor Street, Chicago, Illinois 60612, USA
e-mail: rtassone@uic.edu

Y.-C. Lin
Medical Acupuncture Service, Department of Anesthesiology, Perioperative and Pain Medicine,
Boston Children's Hospital, 300 Longwood Ave., Boston, Massachusetts 02115, USA

Department of Anaesthesia, Harvard Medical School, Boston, Massachusetts, USA
e-mail: yuan-chi.lin@childrens.harvard.edu

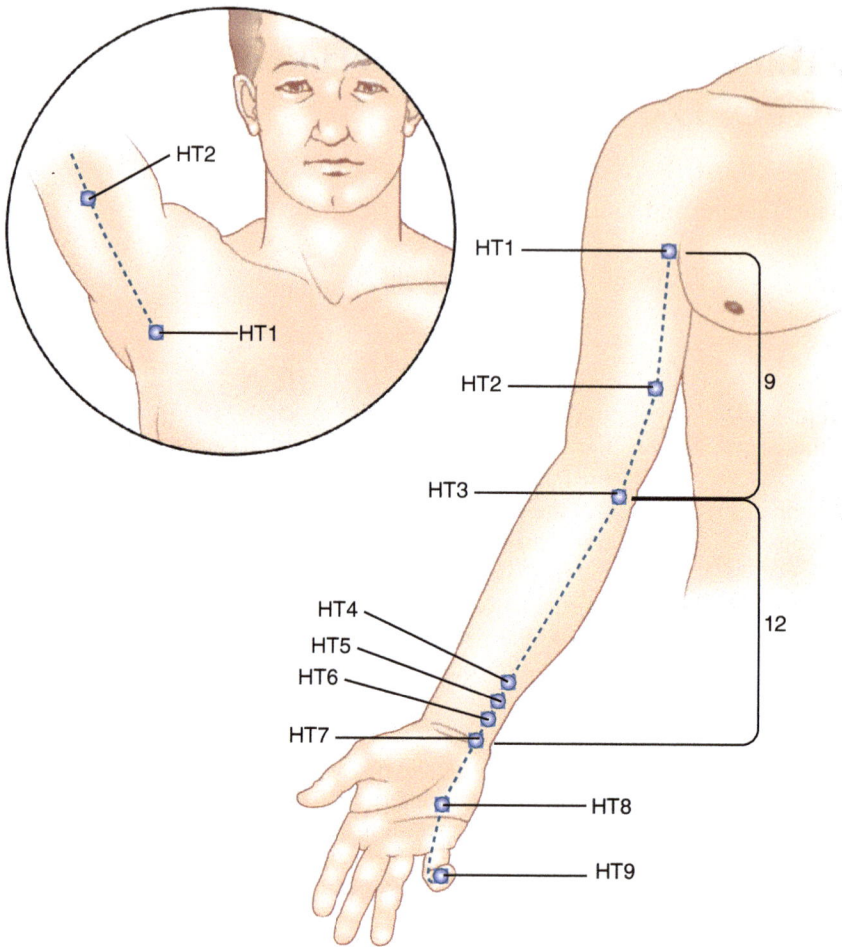

Fig. 14.1 The Hand Shao Yin heart meridian

HT 8 Shaofu 少府	On the palm of hand, in the depression between the fourth and fifth metacarpal bones, proximal to the fifth metacarpophalangeal joint; it also describes the point where the little finger touches the palmar surface when a fist is made.
HT 9 Shaochong 少衝	On the dorsal side of the little finger, 0.1 tsun proximal lateral to the radial side of finger nail bed. (see Fig. 14.1).

Chapter 15
The Hand Tai Yang Small Intestine Meridian
手太陽小腸經穴

Rosalie F. Tassone and Yuan-Chi Lin

SI 1 Shaoze 少澤	On the little finger, 0.1 tsun proximal to the corner of ulnar side of nailbed.
SI 2 Qiangu 前谷	On the little finger, ulnar side of the anterior metacarpophalangeal joint.
SI 3 Houxi 後谿	On the dorsum of the hand, in the depression proximal to the ulnar side of fifth metacarpophalangeal joint.
SI 4 Wangu 腕骨	On the ulnar side of the wrist, at the depression between the fifth metacarpal bone and the triquetral bone.
SI 5 Yanggu 陽谷	On the ulnar side of the wrist, between the triquetral bone and the styloid process.
SI 6 Yanglao 養老	On the dorsal aspect of hand, in the bony cleft on the radial side of the styloid process of the ulna.
SI 7 Zhizheng 支正	On the ulnar side of forearm, 5 tsun above the SI 5 陽谷 Yanggu.
SI 8 Xiaohai 小海	On the dorsal aspect of elbow, in the shallow depression between the olecranon of the ulna and the medial epicondyle of the humerus.
SI 9 Jianzhen 肩貞	On the inferoposterior aspect of the shoulder joint, 1 tsun above the posterior end of the axillary fold.
SI 10 Naoshu 臑俞	On the posterior aspect of shoulder, directly above the SI 9 肩貞 Jianzhen in the depression inferior to the scapular spine.

R. F. Tassone (✉)
Department of Anesthesiology, University of Illinois at Chicago,
1740 West Taylor Street, Chicago, Illinois 60612, USA
e-mail: rtassone@uic.edu

Y.-C. Lin
Medical Acupuncture Service, Department of Anesthesiology, Perioperative and Pain Medicine,
Boston Children's Hospital, 300 Longwood Ave., Boston, Massachusetts 02115, USA

Department of Anaesthesia, Harvard Medical School, Boston, Massachusetts, USA
e-mail: yuan-chi.lin@childrens.harvard.edu

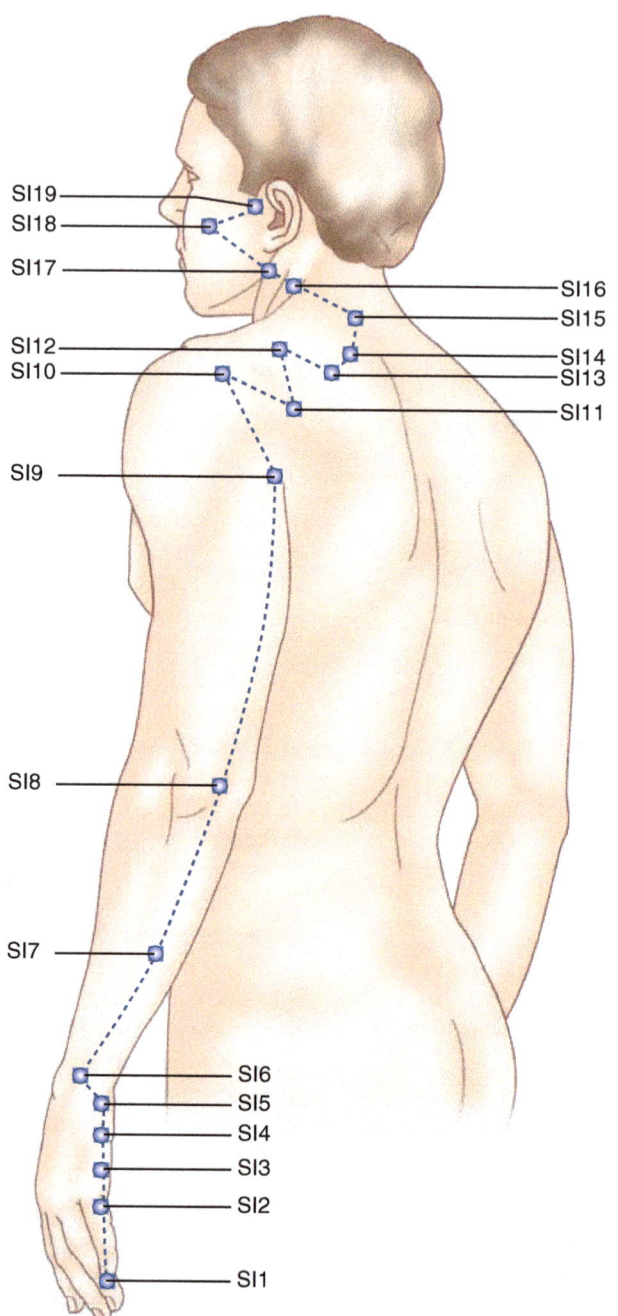

Fig. 15.1 The Hand Tai Yang Small Intestine Meridian

15 The Hand Tai Yang Small Intestine Meridian 手太陽小腸經穴

SI 11 Tianzong 天宗	In the posterior scapula region, in the depression between the upper one third and lower two thirds of the line connecting the midpoint of the spine and lower tip of the scapula.
SI 12 Bingfeng 秉風	On the posterior aspect of the scapula, at the middle of the supraspinous fossa.
SI 13 Quyuan 曲垣	On the medial end of the supraspinous fossa, midway between SI 10 Naoshu 臑俞 and second thoracic vertebra.
SI 14 Jianwaishu 肩外俞	At the level of first spine process of the thoracic vertebrae, 3 tsun lateral to the GV 13 Taodao 陶道.
SI 15 Jianzhongshu 肩中俞	At the level of seventh cervical spine process of the thoracic vertebrae, 2 tsun lateral to the GV 14 Daizhui.
SI 16 Tianchuang 天窗	On the anterior region of the neck, posterior to the sternocleidomastoid muscle at the level of laryngeal prominence.
SI 17 Tianrong 天容	At the posterior-inferior border of the angle of mandible, in the depression on the anterior border of the sternocleidomastoid muscle.
SI 18 Quanliao 顴髎	On the face; inferior to the zygomatic bone, in the depression directly inferior to the outer canthus of the eye.
SI 19 Tinggong 聽宮	In the depression, anterior to the tragus of the ear and behind the posterior border of the condylar process of the mandible (See Fig. 15.1).

Chapter 16
Foot Tai Yang Bladder Meridian 足太陽膀胱經穴

Rosalie F. Tassone and Yuan-Chi Lin

BL 1 Jingming 睛明	On the face, in a depression, just above the inner canthus of the eye.
BL 2 Cuanzhu 攢竹	On the subraorbital notch at the medial end of the eyebrow, directly above the inner canthus of the eye.
BL 3 Meichong 眉衝	On the head, 0.5 cun inside the anterior hairline, directly above BL 2, between GV 24 and BL 4.
BL 4 Qucha 曲差	On the head, 1.5 tsun lateral to GV 24 or 0.5 tsun inside the anterior hairline at the junction of the medial one third and lateral two third's distance between GV 24 and ST 8.
BL 5 Wuchu 五處	On the head, 0.5 tsun behind BL 4 or 1 tsun above the anterior hairline and 1.5 tsun lateral to the anterior midline or 1.5 tsun lateral to GV 23.
BL 6 Chengguang 承光	On the head, 0.5 tsun behind BL 4 or 1 tsun above the anterior hairline and 1.5 tsun lateral to the anterior midline or 1.5 tsun lateral to GV 23.
BL 7 Tongtian 通天	On the head, 1.5 tsun posterior to BL 6 or 4 tsun above the anterior hairline and 1.5 tsun lateral to the anterior midline.
BL 8 Luoque 絡却	On the head, 1.5 tsun posterior to BL 7 or 5.5 tsun above the anterior hairline and 1.5 tsun lateral to the anterior midline.

R. F. Tassone (✉)
Department of Anesthesiology, University of Illinois at Chicago,
1740 West Taylor Street, Chicago, Illinois 60612, USA
e-mail: rtassone@uic.edu

Y.-C. Lin
Medical Acupuncture Service, Department of Anesthesiology, Perioperative and Pain Medicine,
Boston Children's Hospital, 300 Longwood Ave., Boston, Massachusetts 02115, USA

Department of Anaesthesia, Harvard Medical School, Boston, Massachusetts, USA
e-mail: yuan-chi.lin@childrens.harvard.edu

BL9 Yuzhen 玉枕	On the head, 1.3 tsun lateral to GV 17 or 2.5 tsun above the posterior hairline, 1.3 tsun lateral to the posterior midline in a depression in level with GV 17.
BL 10 Tianzhu 天柱	On the posterior region of head, 1.3 tsun lateral to GV 15 in a depression or .5 tsun above the posterior hairline and 1.3 tsun lateral to the posterior midline on the lateral aspect of the trapezius.
BL 11 Dazhu 大抒	On the upper back region, 1.5 tsun lateral to GV 13 in level with T1.
BL 12 Fengmen 風門	On the upper back region, 1.5 tsun lateral to GV line, in level with T2.
BL 13 Feishu 肺俞	On the upper back region, 1.5 tsun lateral to GV 12, in level with T3.
BL 14 Jueyinshu 厥陰俞	On the upper back region, 1.5 tsun lateral to the GV line, in level with T4.
BL 15 Xinshu 心俞	On the upper back region, 1.5 tsun lateral to GV 11, in level with T5.
BL 16 Dushu 督俞	On the upper back region, 1.5 tsun lateral to GV 10, in level with T6.
BL 17 Geshu 隔俞	On the upper back region, 1.5 tsun lateral to GV 9, in level with T7.
BL 18 Ganshu 隔俞	On the upper back region, 1.5 tsun lateral to GV 8, in level with T9.
BL 19 Danshu 胆俞	On the upper back region, 1.5 tsun lateral to GV 7, in level with T10.
BL 20 Pishu 脾俞	On the upper back region, 1.5 tsun lateral to GV 6, in level with T11.
BL 21 weishu 胃俞	On the upper back region, 1.5 tsun lateral to GV line, in level with T12.
BL 22 Sanjiaoshu 三焦俞	In the lumbar region, 1.5 tsun lateral to GV 5, in level with L1.
BL 23 Shenshu 腎俞	In the lumbar region, 1.5 tsun lateral to GV 4, in level with L2.
BL 24 Qihaishu 氣海俞	In the lumbar region, 1.5 tsun lateral to GV line, in level with L3.
BL 25 Dachangshu 大腸俞	In the lumbar region, 1.5 tsun lateral to GV 3, in level with L4.
BL 26 Guanyuanshu 關元俞	In the lumbar region, 1.5 tsun lateral to GV line, in level with L5.
BL 27 Xinochaogshu 小腸俞	In the sacral region, 1.5 tsun lateral to GV line, in level with 1st posterior sacral foramen.
BL 28 Pangguangshu 膀胱俞	In the sacral region, 1.5 tsun lateral to GV line, in level with 2nd posterior sacral foramen.
BL 29 Zhonglushu 中膂俞	In the sacral region, 1.5 tsun lateral to the GV line, in level with the 3rd posterior sacral foramen.

BL 30 Baihuanshu 白環俞	In the sacral region, 1.5 tsun lateral to the GV line, in level with the 4th posterior sacral foramen.
BL 31 Shangliao 上髎	On the sacrum at the midpoint of the PSIS and the posterior midline, in level with the 1st posterior sacral foramen.
BL 32 Ciliao 次髎	On the sacrum medial and inferior to the PSIS, in level with the 2nd posterior sacral foramen.
BL 33 Zhongliao 中髎	On the sacrum medial and inferior to BL 32, in level with the 3rd posterior sacral foramen.
BL 34 Xialiao 下髎	On the sacrum lateral to GV 2, in level with the 4th posterior sacral foramen.
BL 35 Huiyang 會陽	In the buttock, 0.5 tsun lateral to the GV line on either side of the tip of the coccyx bone.
BL 36 Chengfu 承扶	In the prone position, on posterior side of the thigh at the midpoint of the inferior gluteal crease.
BL 37 Yinmen 殷門	On the posterior aspect of thigh, 6 tsun below BL 36 on a line joining BL 36 and BL 40.
BL 38 Fuxi 浮郄	With the knee slightly bent, 1 tsun above BL 39 on the medial side of the tendon of biceps femoris.
BL 39 Weiyans 委陽	On the posterolateral aspect of knee, lateral to BL 40 on the medial border of the tendon of biceps femoris.
BL 40 Weizhong 委中	On the posterior aspect of knee, midpoint of the transverse crease of the popliteal fossa, between the tendons of biceps femoris and semitendinosus.
BL 41 Fufen 附分	In the upper back region, 3 tsun lateral to the GV line, in level with T2, on the spinal border of the scapula.
BL 42 Pohu 魄戶	In the upper back region, 3 tsun lateral to GV 12, in level with T3, on the spinal border of the scapula.
BL 43 Gaohuans 膏肓	In the upper back region, 3 tsun lateral to the GV line, in level with T4.
BL 44 Shentang 神堂	In the upper back region, 3 tsun lateral to GV 11, in level with T5.
BL 45 Yixi 譩譆	In the upper back region, 3 tsun lateral to GV 10, in level with T6.
BL 46 Geguan 隔關	In the upper back region, 3 tsun lateral to GV 9, in level with T7.
BL 47 Hunmen 魂門	In the upper back region, 3 tsun lateral to GV 8, in level with T9.
BL 48 Yanggang 陽網	In the upper back region, 3 tsun lateral to GV 7, in level with T10.
BL 49 Yishe 意舍	In the upper back region, 3 tsun lateral to GV 6, in level with T11.
BL 50 Weicang 胃倉	In the upper back region, 3 tsun lateral to the GV line, in level with T12.
BL 51 Huangmen 肓門	In the lumbar region, 3 tsun lateral to GV 5, in level with L1.

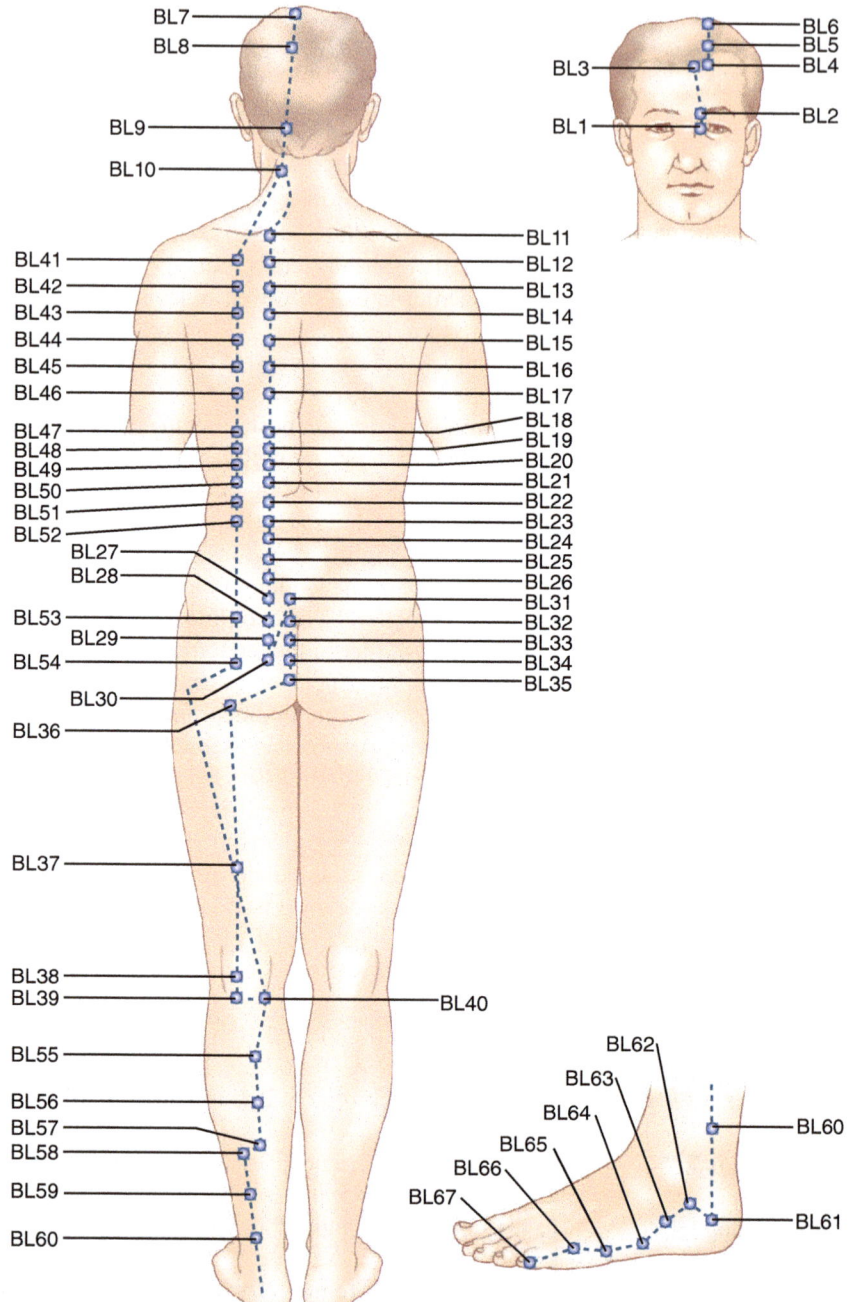

Fig. 16.1 Foot Tai Yang Bladder Meridian

16 Foot Tai Yang Bladder Meridian 足太陽膀胱經穴

BL 52 Zhishi 志室	In the lumbar region, 3 tsun lateral to GV 4, in level with L2.
BL 53 Baohuang 胞盲	On the buttock region, 3 tsun lateral to the medial sacral crest, in level with the 2nd posterior sacral foramen.
BL 54 Zhibian 秩邊	On the buttock region, 3 tsun lateral to the GV line, in level with the 4th sacral foramen.
BL 55 Heyang 合陽	On the posterior aspect of the leg, 2 tsun directly below BL 40 between the medial and lateral heads of the gastrocnemius, on a line joining BL 40–BL 57.
BL 56 Chengjin 承筋	On the posterior aspect of the leg, 5 tsun below BL 40 on the line connecting BL 40–BL 57, midway between BL 55 and BL 57 in the center of the belly of the gastrocnemius.
BL 57 Chengshan 承山	On the posterolateral aspect of the leg, 8 tsun below BL 40 in a pointed depression below the gastrocnemius when leg is stretched or heel is lifted.
BL 58 Feiyang 飛揚	On the posterolateral aspect of the leg, 7 tsun directly above BL 60 on the posterior border of the fibula about 1 tsun lateral and inferior to BL 57.
BL 59 Fuyang 附陽	On the posterolateral aspect of the leg, 3 tsun directly proximal to BL 60.
BL 60 Kunlun 崑崙	On the posterolateral aspect of ankle, in a depression between the tip of the external malleolus and the Achilles tendon.
BL 61 Pushen 僕參	On the lateral aspect of foot, posterior and Inferior to the external malleolus, directly below BL 60, lateral to the calcaneum at the junction of the dorsal and plantar skin.
BL 62 Shenmai 申脈	On the lateral aspect of foot, in a depression directly below the external malleolus.
BL 63 Jinmen 金門	On the lateral side of the foot, directly below the anterior border of the external malleolus, on the lower border of the cuboid bone.
BL 64 Jinggu 京骨	On the lateral aspect of foot, below the tuberosity of the 5th metatarsal bone at the junction of the dorsal and plantar skin.
BL 65 Shugu 束骨	On the lateral aspect of foot, in the depression, posterior to the 5th metatarsophalangeal joint at the junction of the dorsal and plantar skin.
BL 66 Zutonggu 足通谷	On the little toe, distal and lateral to the 5th metatarsophalangeal joint at the junction of the dorsal and plantar skin.
BL 67 Zhiyin 至陰	On the little toe, 0.1 tsun posterior to the corner of the nail on the lateral side of the little toenail. (See Fig. 16.1)

Chapter 17
Foot Shao Yin Kidney Meridian 足少陰腎經穴

Rosalie F. Tassone and Yuan-Chi Lin

KI 1 Yongquan 湧泉	On the sole of the foot, in the depression when foot in plantar flexion, at the junction of the anterior one third and posterior two third of the line connecting the base of the second and third toes with the heel.
KI 2 Rangu 然谷	Anterior and inferior to the medial malleolus in a depression on the lower border of the tuberosity of the navicular bone.
KI 3 Taixi 太溪	On the posteromedial aspect of ankle, in the depression midway between the tip of the medial malleolus and the attachment of the Achilles tendon.
KI 4 Dazhong 大鐘	On the medial aspect of foot, posterior and inferior to the medial malleolus in a depression anterior to the medial attachment of the Achilles tendon.
KI 5 Shuiquan 水泉	On the medial aspect of foot, 1 tsun directly below KI 3 in a depression on the medial side of the tuberosity of the calcaneus.
KI 6 Zhaohai 照海	On the medial aspect of foot, in a depression below the tip of the medial malleolus.
KI 7 Fuliu 復溜	On the posteromedial aspect of foot, 2 tsun above KI 3 on the anterior border of the Achilles tendon.

R. F. Tassone (✉)
Department of Anesthesiology, University of Illinois at Chicago,
1740 West Taylor Street, Chicago, Illinois 60612, USA
e-mail: rtassone@uic.edu

Y.-C. Lin
Medical Acupuncture Service, Department of Anesthesiology, Perioperative and Pain Medicine,
Boston Children's Hospital, 300 Longwood Ave., Boston, Massachusetts 02115, USA

Department of Anaesthesia, Harvard Medical School, Boston, Massachusetts, USA
e-mail: yuan-chi.lin@childrens.harvard.edu

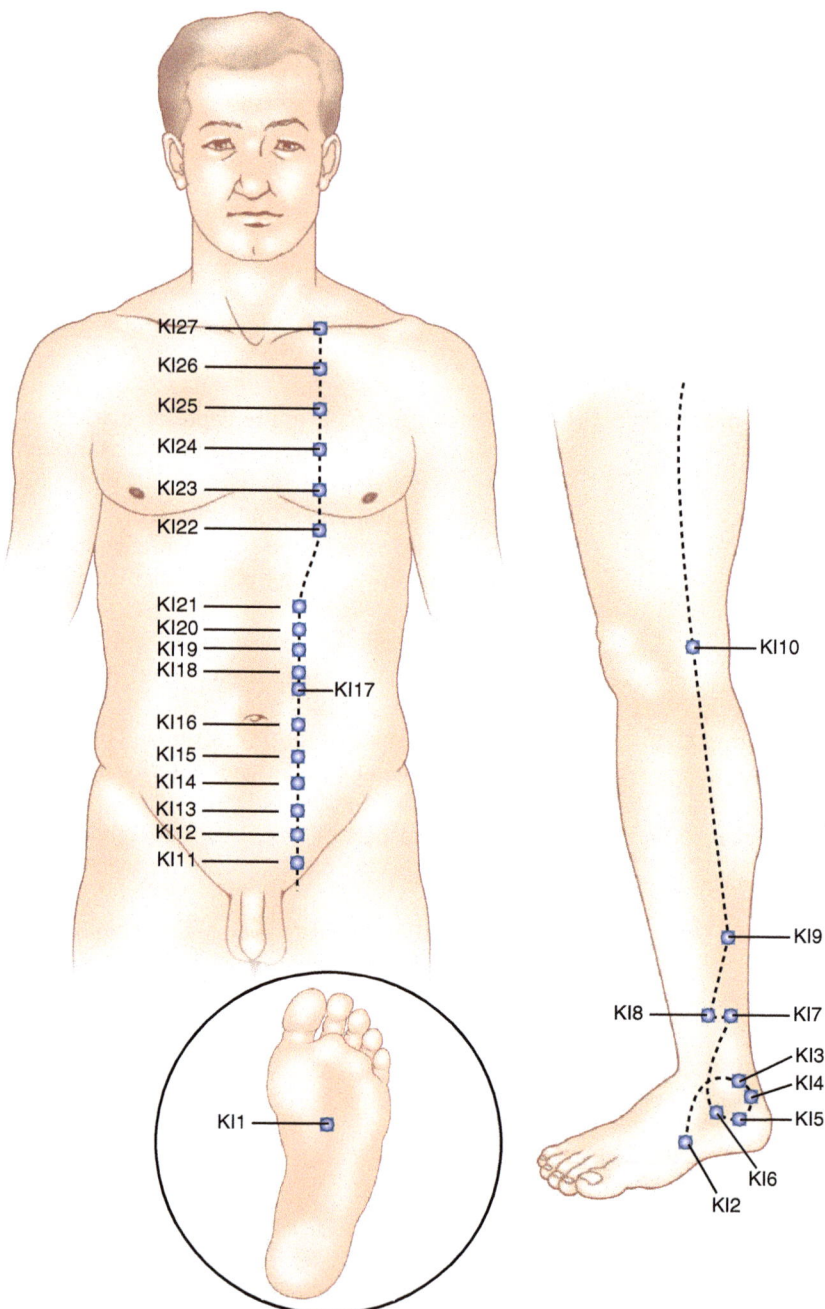

Fig. 17.1 Foot Shao Yin Kidney Meridian

17 Foot Shao Yin Kidney Meridian 足少陰腎經穴

KI 8 Jiaoxin 交信	On the medial aspect of leg, 0.5 tsun anterior to KI 7, 2 tsun above KI 3 posterior to the medial border of the tibia.
KI 9 Zhubin 築賓	On the posteromedial aspect of the leg, 5 tsun above KI 3 on the line drawn from KI 3 to KI 10 at the lower end of the belly of the gastrocnemius muscle.
KI 10 Yingu 陰谷	On the posteromedial side of the knee joint between the tendons of semitendinosus and semimembranosus.
KI 11 Henggu 橫骨	On the lower abdomen, 5 tsun below umbilicus, 0.5 tsun lateral to CV 2.
KI 12 Dahe 大赫	On the lower abdomen, 4 tsun below umbilicus, 0.5 tsun lateral to CV 3.
KI 13 Qixue 氣穴	On the lower abdomen, 3 tsun below umbilicus, 0.5 tsun lateral to CV 4.
KI 14 Siman 四滿	On the lower abdomen, 1 tsun below umbilicus, 0.5 tsun lateral to CV 5.
KI 15 Zhonszhu 中注	On the lower abdomen, 1 tsun below umbilicus, 0.5 tsun lateral to CV 7.
KI 16 Huangshu 盲俞	On the lower abdomen, 0.5 tsun below umbilicus.
KI 17 Shangqu 商曲	On the upper abdomen, 2 tsun superior to the umbilicus, 5 tsun lateral to CV 10.
KI 18 Shiguan 石關	On the upper abdomen, 3 tsun superior to the umbilicus, 0.5 tsun lateral to CV 11.
KI 19 Yindu 陰都	On the upper abdomen, 4 tsun superior to the umbilicus, 0.5 tsun lateral to CV 12.
KI 20 Futonggu 腹通谷	On the upper abdomen, 5 tsun superior to the umbilicus, 0.5 tsun lateral to CV 13.
KIU 21 Youmen 幽門	On the upper abdomen, 6 tsun superior to the umbilicus, 0.5 tsun lateral to CV 14.
KI 22 Bulang 步廊	In the anterior thorax region, 5th intercostal space, 2 tsun lateral to CV 16.
KI 23 Shenfeng 神封	In the anterior thorax region; 4th intercostal space CS 2 tsun lateral to CV 17.
KI 24 Lingxu 靈墟	In the anterior thorax region; 3rd intercostal space, 2 tsun lateral to CV 18.
KI 25 Shencang 神藏	In the anterior thorax region; 2nd intercostal space, 2 tsun lateral to CV 19.
KI 26 Yuzhong 彧中	In the anterior thoracic region; 1st intercostal space, 2 tsun lateral to CV 20.
KI 27 Shufu 俞府	In the anterior thoracic region, in a depression on the lower border of the clavicle, 2 tsun lateral to the anterior median CV line. (See Fig 17.1)

Chapter 18
Hand Jue Yin Pericardium Meridian
手厥陰心包經穴

Lynn M. Rusy and Yuan-Chi Lin

PC 1 Tianchi	In the anterior chest region, fourth intercostal space, 5 tsun lateral to the anterior median line
PC 2 Tianquan	In the anterior aspect of arm, 2 tsun inferior to the anterior axillary fold, between the two heads of biceps brachii muscle
PC 3 Quze	In the anterior aspect of elbow, at the transverse cubital crease, medial to the biceps brachii tendon
PC 4 Ximen	In the anterior aspect of forearm, 5 tsun proximal to the transverse crease of the wrist, between the tendons of the palmaris longus and the flexor carpi radialis
PC 5 Jianshi	In the anterior aspect of forearm, 3 tsun proximal to the transverse crease of the wrist, between the tendons of the palmaris longus and the flexor carpi radialis
PC 6 Neiguan	In the anterior aspect of forearm, 2 tsun proximal to the transverse crease of the wrist, between the tendons of the palmaris longus and the flexor carpi radialis
PC 7 Daling	In the anterior aspect of forearm, in the depression on the middle of the transverse crease of the wrist, between the tendons of the palmaris longus and the flexor carpi radialis

---

L. M. Rusy (✉)
Department of Anesthesia, Children's Hospital of Wisconsin,
9000 West Wisconsin Avenue, MS792, Milwaukee, Wisconsin 53221, USA
e-mail: lrusy@mcw.edu

Y.-C. Lin
Medical Acupuncture Service, Department of Anesthesiology, Perioperative and Pain Medicine,
Boston Children's Hospital, 300 Longwood Ave., Boston, Massachusetts 02115, USA

Department of Anaesthesia, Harvard Medical School, Boston, Massachusetts, USA
e-mail: yuan-chi.lin@childrens.harvard.edu

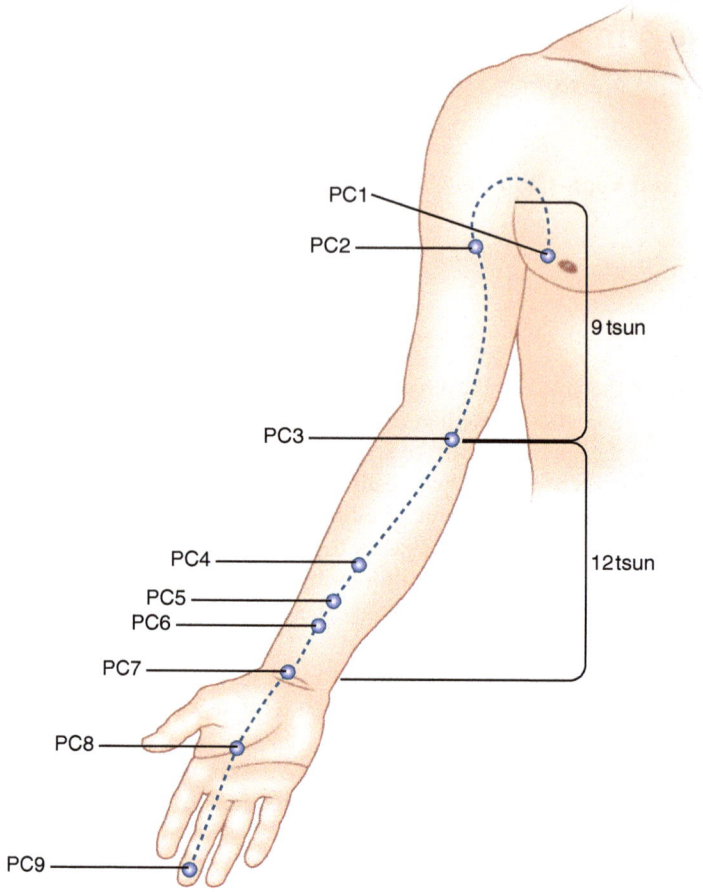

Fig. 18.1 The Hand Jue Yin pericardium meridian

PC 8 Laogong   On the palm of the hand, between second and third metacarpal bones, proximal to the metacarpophalangeal joints
PC 9 Zhongchong On the middle finger, at the midpoint of the tip of middle finger (see Fig. 18.1)

Chapter 19
Hand Sho Yang Triple Energizer Meridian
手少陽三焦經穴

Lynn M. Rusy and Yuan-Chi Lin

TE 1 Guanchong 關衝	On the ulnar side of the ring finger, 0.1 tsun lateral to the corner of the nail bed
TE 2 Yemen 液門	On the dorsum of the hand, 0.5 tsun proximal to the margin of web between the ring and small finger
TE 3 Zhongzhu 中渚	On the dorsum of the hand, between the fourth and fifth metacarpals in a deep depression proximal to the metacarpophalangeal joint
TE 4 Yangchi 陽池	On the dorsum of the wrist, at the depression of the transverse crease, ulnar to the tendon of extensor digit rum communis muscle
TE 5 Waiguan 外關	On the dorsum of forearm, 2 tsun proximal to the dorsal wrist crease, between ulnar and radius
TE 6 Zhigou 支溝	On the dorsum of forearm, 3 tsun proximal to the dorsal wrist crease, between ulnar and radius
TE 7 Huizong 會宗	On the dorsum of forearm, 3 tsun proximal to the dorsal wrist crease, on the radial side of ulnar
TE 8 Sanyangluo 三陽絡	On the dorsum of forearm, 4 tsun proximal to the dorsal wrist crease, between ulnar and radius
TE 9 Sidu 四瀆	On the dorsum of forearm, 5 tsun proximal to the dorsal wrist crease, between ulnar and radius
TE 10 Tianjing 天井	On the dorsum of the elbow, 1 tsun proximal to the prominence of the olecranon, in the depression

L. M. Rusy (✉)
Department of Anesthesia, Children's Hospital of Wisconsin,
9000 West Wisconsin Avenue MS792, Milwaukee, Wisconsin 53221, USA
e-mail: lrusy@mcw.edu

Y.-C. Lin
Medical Acupuncture Service, Department of Anesthesiology, Perioperative and Pain Medicine,
Boston Children's Hospital, 300 Longwood Ave., Boston, Massachusetts 02115, USA

Department of Anaesthesia, Harvard Medical School, Boston, Massachusetts, USA
e-mail: yuan-chi.lin@childrens.harvard.edu

Fig. 19.1 The Hand Sho Yang triple energizer meridian

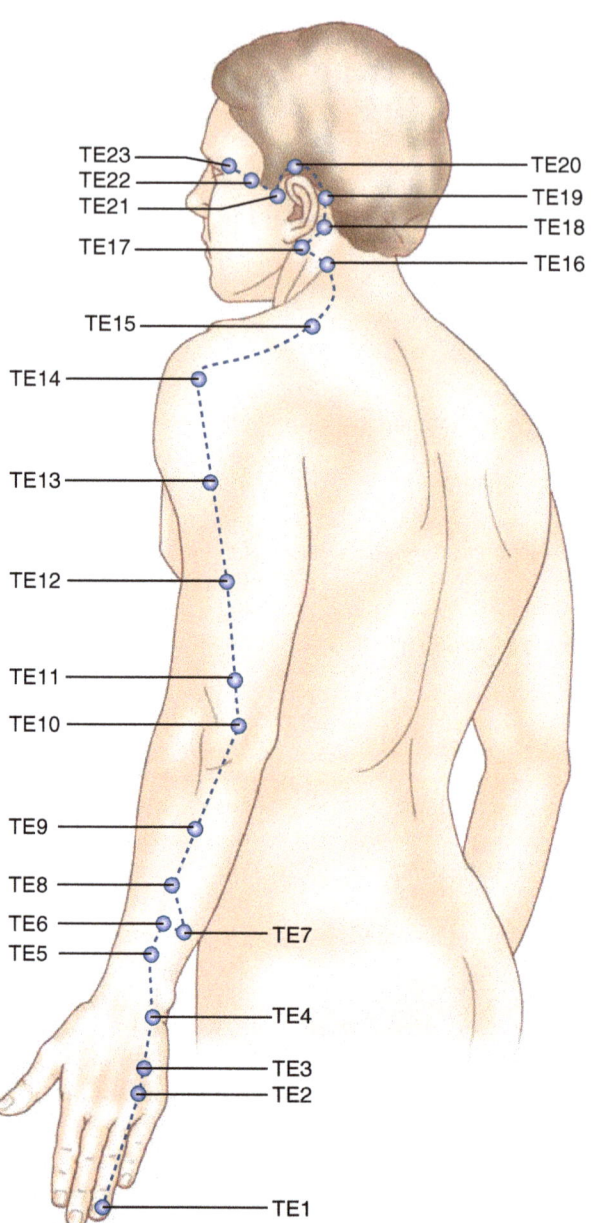

| TE 11 Qinglengyuan 清冷淵 | On the dorsum of the arm, 2 tsun proximal to the prominence of the olecranon |
| TE 12 Xiaoluo 消濼 | On the dorsum of arm, 5 tsun proximal to the prominence of the olecranon, midway between TE 11 and TE 13 |

19 Hand Sho Yang Triple Energizer Meridian 手少陽三焦經穴

TE 13 Naohui 臑會	On the dorsum of arm, 3 tsun below the TE 14 肩髎 Jianliao, at the posterior border of the deltoid muscle
TE 14 Jianliao 肩髎	On the great depression at the posteroinferior part of acromion
TE 15 Tianliao 天髎	On the superior angle of scapula, midway between acromion and GV 14
TE 16 Tianyu 天牖	Posterior and inferior to the mastoid process, over the posterior border of the sternocleidomastoid muscle
TE 17 Yifeng 翳風	Behind the ear lobe, in the depression between the mastoid process and the mandible
TE 18 Chimai 瘈脈	At the center of mastoid process
TE 19 Luxi 顱息	Posterior to the root of ear, at the junction of upper and middle third of the curve formed by TE 17 and TE 20
TE 20 Jiaosun 角孫	On the temple hairline directly superior to the ear apex
TE 21 Ermen 耳門	On the anterior of the ear, in the depression anterior to the supratragic notch and condyloid process of the mandible when the mouth is open
TE 22 Erheliao 耳和髎	Anterior to the upper auricular root and superior to TE 21
TE 23 Sizhukong 絲竹空	On the depression at the lateral end of eyebrow (see Fig. 19.1)

Chapter 20
Foot Shao Yang Gall Bladder Meridian
足少陽膽經穴

Lynn M. Rusy and Yuan-Chi Lin

GB 1 Tongziliao 瞳子髎	On the head, 0.5 tsun lateral to the external canthus of the eye
GB 2 Tinghui 聽會	On the side of face anterior to the ear, anterior to the intertragic notch, in a depression
GB 3 Shangguan 上關	On the side of face anterior to the ear, at the upper border of the zygomatic arch
GB 4 Hanyan 頷厭	On the side of face in the temporal region, a quarter of the distance between ST 8 and GB 7
GB 5 Xuanlu 懸顱	On the side of face in the temporal region, at the midway between ST 8 Touwei 頭維 and GB 7 Qubin 曲鬢
GB 6 Xuanli 懸厘	On the side of face in the temporal region, at the midway between GB 5 Xuanlu 懸顱 and GB 7 Qubin 曲鬢
GB 7 Qubin 曲鬢	On the side of face anterior to the apex of the ear, 1 tsun anterior to the TE 20 Jiaosun 角孫.
GB 8 Shuaigu 率谷	On the side of face in the temporal region, superior to the auricle and 1.5 tsun superior to the hairline
GB 9 Tianchong 天衝	On the side of face in the temporal region, posterior and superior to the auricle, 0.5 tsun posterior to GB 8 率谷 Shuaigu
GB 10 Fubai 浮白	Posterior to the auricle, on the posterosuperior aspect of mastoid process, in the midline between GB 9 Tianchong 天衝 and GB 11 Touqiaoyin 頭窍陰

L. M. Rusy (✉)
Department of Anesthesia, Children's Hospital of Wisconsin,
9000 West Wisconsin Avenue MS792, Milwaukee, Wisconsin 53221, USA
e-mail: lrusy@mcw.edu

Y.-C. Lin
Medical Acupuncture Service, Department of Anesthesiology, Perioperative and Pain Medicine,
Boston Children's Hospital, 300 Longwood Ave., Boston, Massachusetts 02115, USA

Department of Anaesthesia, Harvard Medical School, Boston, Massachusetts, USA
e-mail: yuan-chi.lin@childrens.harvard.edu

GB 11 Touqiaoyin 頭窍陰	Posterior to the auricle, 1 tsun inferior to GB 10 Fubai 浮白
GB 12 Wangu 完骨	Posterior to the auricle, in the depression posterior and inferior to the mastoid process
GB 13 Benshen 本神	On the forehead, 0.5 tsun superior to the hairline, 3 tsun lateral to the anterior median line, directly above the outer canthus
GB 14 Yangbai 陽白	On the forehead, 1 tsun above the midpoint of eyebrow
GB 15 Toulinqi 頭臨泣	On the forehead, 0.5 tsun within the anterior hairline, directly superior to the center of the eye
GB 16 Muchuang 目窗	On the forehead, 1.5 tsun directly superior to GB 15 Toulinqi 頭臨泣
GB 17 Zhengyins 正營	Near the top of the head, 1 tsun directly superior to GB 16 Muchuang 目窗
GB 18 Chegling 承靈	On the posterior aspect of head, 1.5 tsun posterior to GB 17 Zhengyins 正營, on the line between GB 15 Toulinqi 頭臨泣 and GB 20 Fengchi 風池
GB 19 Naokong 腦空	On the posterior aspect of head, 1.5 tsun posterior to GB 18 Chegling 承靈, on the line between GB 15 Toulinqi 頭臨泣 and GB 20 Fengchi 風池
GB 20 Fengchi 風池	On the posterior aspect of the neck, depression between the origins of sternocleidomastoid and the trapezius muscles
GB 21 Jianjing 肩井	On the shoulder, midway between GV 14 大椎 Daizhui and acromion
GB 22 Yuanye 淵腋	On the lateral thoracic region, in the fourth intercostals space, on the mid-axillary line
GB 23 Zhejin 輒筋	On the lateral thoracic region, in the fourth intercostals space, 1 tsun anterior to GB 22 淵腋 Yuanye
GB 24 Jihyueh 日月	On the anterolateral chest region, seventh intercostals space, 4 tsun lateral to the anterior median line
GB 25 Jingmen 京門	On the lateral abdomen, inferior border of the free 12th ribs
GB 26 Daimai 帶脈	On the lateral abdomen, inferior to the free 11th ribs, at the same level of umbilicus
GB 27 Wushu 五樞	On the lower abdomen, at the level of 3 tsun inferior to the center of umbilicus, medial to the anterior superior iliac spine
GB 28 Weidao 維道	On the lower abdomen, 0.5 tsun medioinferior to GB 27 五樞 Wushu
GB 29 Juliao 居髎	On the buttock region, midpoint between anterior superior iliac spine and greater trochanter
GB 30 Huantiao 環跳	On the buttock region, lateral one third and medical two thirds of the line connecting the prominence of the greater trochanter and sacral hiatus

20 Foot Shao Yang Gall Bladder Meridian 足少陽膽經穴

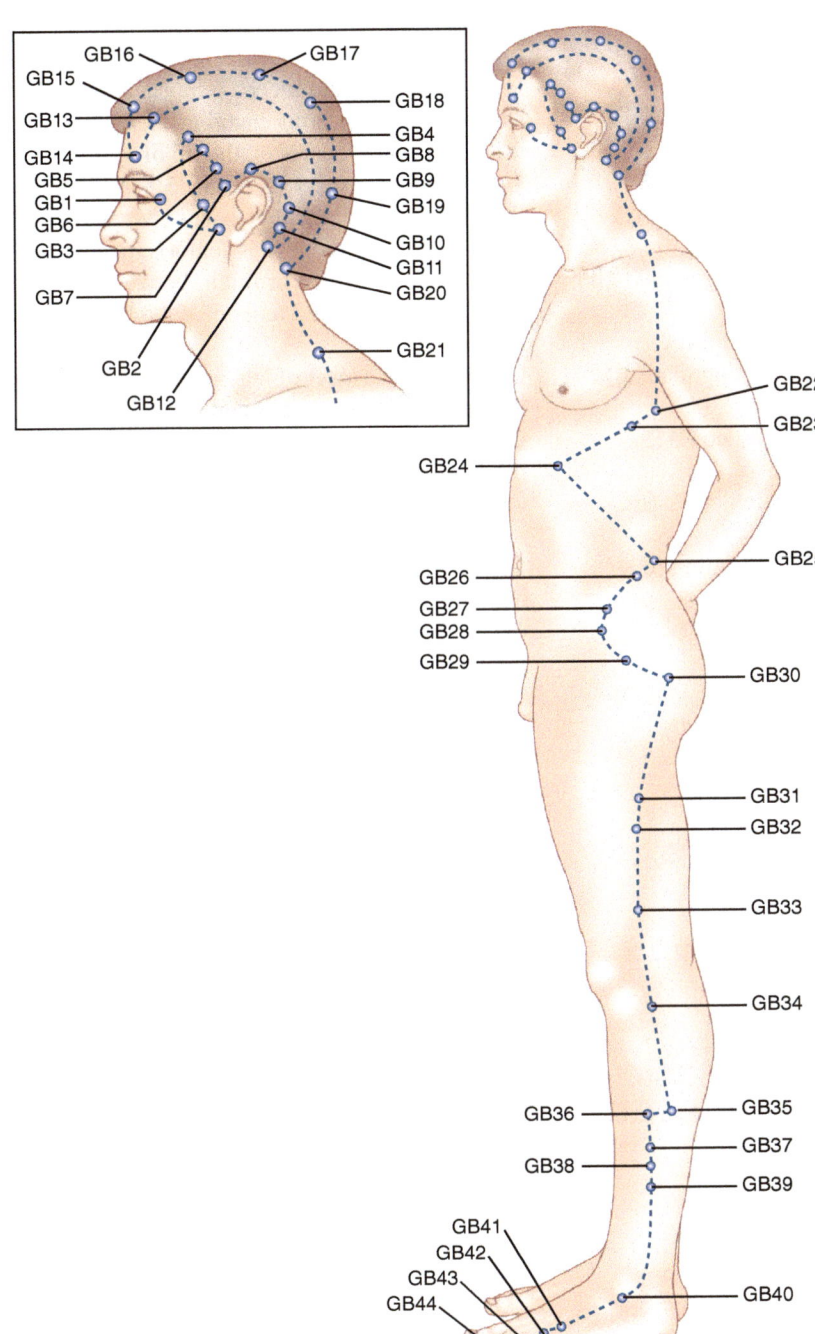

Fig. 20.1 The Foot Shao Yang gall bladder meridian

GB 31 Fengshi 風市	On the lateral side of thigh, 7 tsun superior to the transverse popliteal crease, between the vastus lateralis muscle and biceps femoris muscle. When standing up with arms hanging along the side of thigh, the point locates on the tip of middle finger
GB 32 Zhongdu 中瀆	On the lateral aspect of thigh, 5 tsun superior to the transverse popliteal crease, between the vastus lateralis muscle and biceps femoris muscle
GB 33 Xiyangguan 膝陽關	On the lateral aspect of thigh, between the lateral condyle of femur and tendon of the biceps muscle of femur
GB 34 Yanglingquan 陽陵泉	On the lateral aspect of leg, anterior and inferior to the head of fibula in the great depression
GB 35 Yangjiao 陽交	On the lateral aspect of leg, 7 tsun above the lateral malleolus, in the posterior border of fibula
GB 36 Waichiou 外丘	On the lateral aspect of leg, 7 tsun above the lateral malleolus, in the anterior border of fibula
GB 37 Guangming 光明	On the lateral aspect of leg, 5 tsun above the lateral malleolus, in the anterior border of fibula
GB 38 Yangfu 陽輔	On the lateral aspect of leg, 4 tsun above the lateral malleolus, in the posterior border of fibula
GB 39 Xuanzhong 懸鐘	On the lateral aspect of leg, 3 tsun above the lateral malleolus, in the posterior border of fibula
GB 40 Qiuxu 丘墟	On the dorsum aspect of foot, anterior inferior to the lateral malleolus, on the depression lateral of the tendon the long extensor muscle
GB 41 Zulinqi 足臨泣	On the dorsum aspect of foot, in the depression distal to the junction of the fourth and fifth metatarsal bones
GB 42 Diwuhui 地五會	On the dorsum aspect of foot, in the depression proximal to the fourth metatarsophalangeal joint, between the fourth and fifth metatarsal bones
GB 43 Jiaxi 俠谿	On the dorsum aspect of foot, between the fourth and fifth toes, proximal to the margin of the web
GB 44 Zuqiaoyin 足竅陰	On the lateral side of fourth toe, about 0.1 tsun proximal to the corner of the nail bed (see Fig. 20.1)

Chapter 21
Foot Jun Yin Liver Meridian 足厥陰肝經穴

Lynn M. Rusy and Yuan-Chi Lin

LR 1 Dadun 大敦	On the lateral side of great toe, about 0.1 tsun proximal to the corner of the nail bed.
LR 2 Xingjian 行間	On the dorsal aspect of the foot, 0.5 tsun proximal to the web margin between the first and second metatarsophalangeal joint.
LR 3 Taichong 太衝	On the dorsal aspect of the foot, 2 tsun proximal to the web margin between the first and second metatarsals.
LR 4 Zhongfeng 中封	On the dorsal aspect of foot, 1 tsun anterior to the medial malleolus, between the tendon of extensor hallucis longus and tibialis anterior muscles.
LR 5 Ligou 蠡溝	On the medical aspect tibia, in the depression 5 tsun above the medial malleolus.
LR 6 Zhongdu 中都	On the medical aspect tibia, in the depression 7 tsun above the medial malleolus.
LR 7 Xiguan 膝關	On the medial aspect of proximal tibia, inferior to the medial condyle of the tibia.
LR 8 Ququan 曲泉	On the medial portion of popliteal fossa, posterior to the medial condyle of the tibia and anterior to the semimembranosus muscle.
LR 9 Yinbao 陰包	On the medial aspect of thigh, 4 tsun above the medial condyle of femur, between the vastus medialis muscle and Sartorius muscles.

L. M. Rusy (✉)
Department of Anesthesia, Children's Hospital of Wisconsin,
9000 West Wisconsin Avenue MS792, Milwaukee, Wisconsin 53221, USA
e-mail: lrusy@mcw.edu

Y.-C. Lin
Medical Acupuncture Service, Department of Anesthesiology, Perioperative and Pain Medicine,
Boston Children's Hospital, 300 Longwood Ave., Boston, Massachusetts 02115, USA

Department of Anaesthesia, Harvard Medical School, Boston, Massachusetts, USA
e-mail: yuan-chi.lin@childrens.harvard.edu

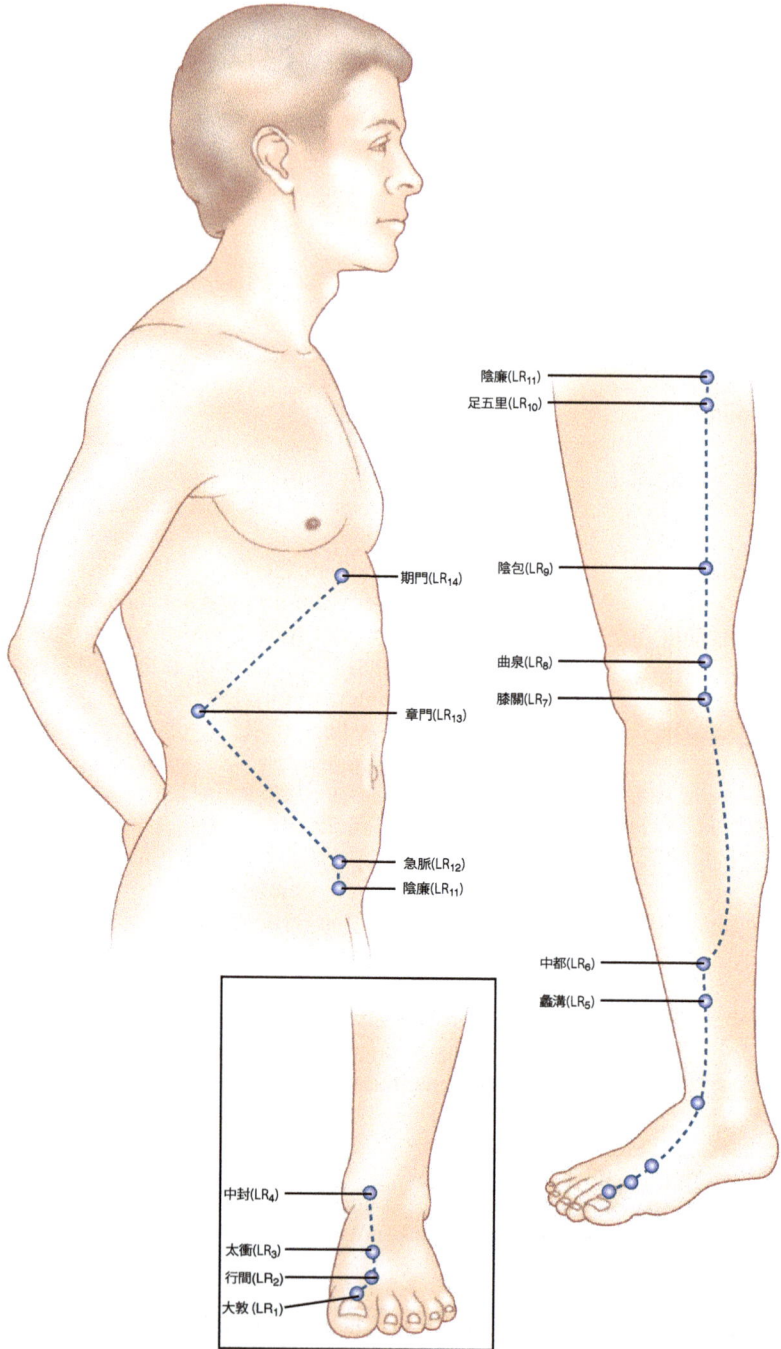

Fig. 21.1 The Foot Jun Yin Liver Meridian

LR 10 Zuwuli 足五里		On the medial aspect of thigh, 3 tsun inferior the ST 30 Qichong 氣衝, lateral to the adductor muscle.
LR 11 Yinlian 陰廉		On the medial aspect of thigh, 2 tsun inferior and 0. tsun lateral to the ST 30.
LR 12 Jimai 急脈		In the groin region, 2.5 tsun lateral to the center of pubic symphysis.
LR 13 Zhangmen 章門		At the level of 11th floating rib, on the anterior axillary line.
LR 14 Qimen 期門		On the anterior thoracic region, in the sixth intercostals space, 4 tsun lateral to the anterior median line (see Fig. 21.1).

Chapter 22
Conception Vessel 任脈經穴

Yuan-Chi Lin and Lynn M. Rusy

CV 1 Huiyin 會陰	Between the anus and root of external genitalia.
CV 2 Qugu 曲骨	At the midline of pubic symphysis superior border.
CV 3 Zhongji 中極	At the anterior mid abdomen, 4 tsun below the umbilicus.
CV 4 Guanyuan 關元	At the anterior mid abdomen, 3 tsun below the umbilicus.
CV 5 Shimen 石門	At the anterior mid abdomen, 2 tsun below the umbilicus.
CV 6 Qihai 氣海	At the anterior mid abdomen, 1.5 tsun below the umbilicus.
CV 7 Yinjiao 陰交	At the anterior mid abdomen, 1 tsun below the umbilicus.
CV 8 Shenque 神闕	At the center of umbilicus.
CV 9 Shuifen 水分	At the anterior mid abdomen, 1 tsun above the umbilicus.
CV 10 Xiawan 下脘	At the anterior mid abdomen, 2 tsun above the umbilicus.
CV 11 Jianli 建里	At the anterior mid abdomen, 3 tsun above the umbilicus.
CV 12 Zhongwan 中脘	At the anterior mid abdomen, 4 tsun above the umbilicus.
CV 13 Shangwan 上脘	At the anterior mid abdomen, 5 tsun above the umbilicus.
CV 14 Juque 巨闕	At the anterior mid abdomen, 6 tsun above the umbilicus.
CV 15 Jiuwei 鳩尾	At the anterior mid abdomen, 7 tsun above the umbilicus, below the xyphoid process.
CV 16 Zhongting 中庭	At the midline anterior chest, at the level of fifth intercostals.
CV 17 Dhozhong 膻中	At the midline anterior chest, between the nipples; at the level of fourth intercostals.
CV 18 Yutang 玉堂	At the midline anterior chest, at the level of third intercostals.

Y.-C. Lin (✉)
Medical Acupuncture Service, Department of Anesthesiology, Perioperative and Pain Medicine,
Boston Children's Hospital, 300 Longwood Ave., Boston, Massachusetts 02115, USA

Department of Anaesthesia, Harvard Medical School, Boston, Massachusetts, USA
e-mail: yuan-chi.lin@childrens.harvard.edu

L. M. Rusy
Department of Anesthesia, Children's Hospital of Wisconsin,
9000 West Wisconsin Avenue MS792, Milwaukee, Wisconsin 53221, USA
e-mail: lrusy@mcw.edu

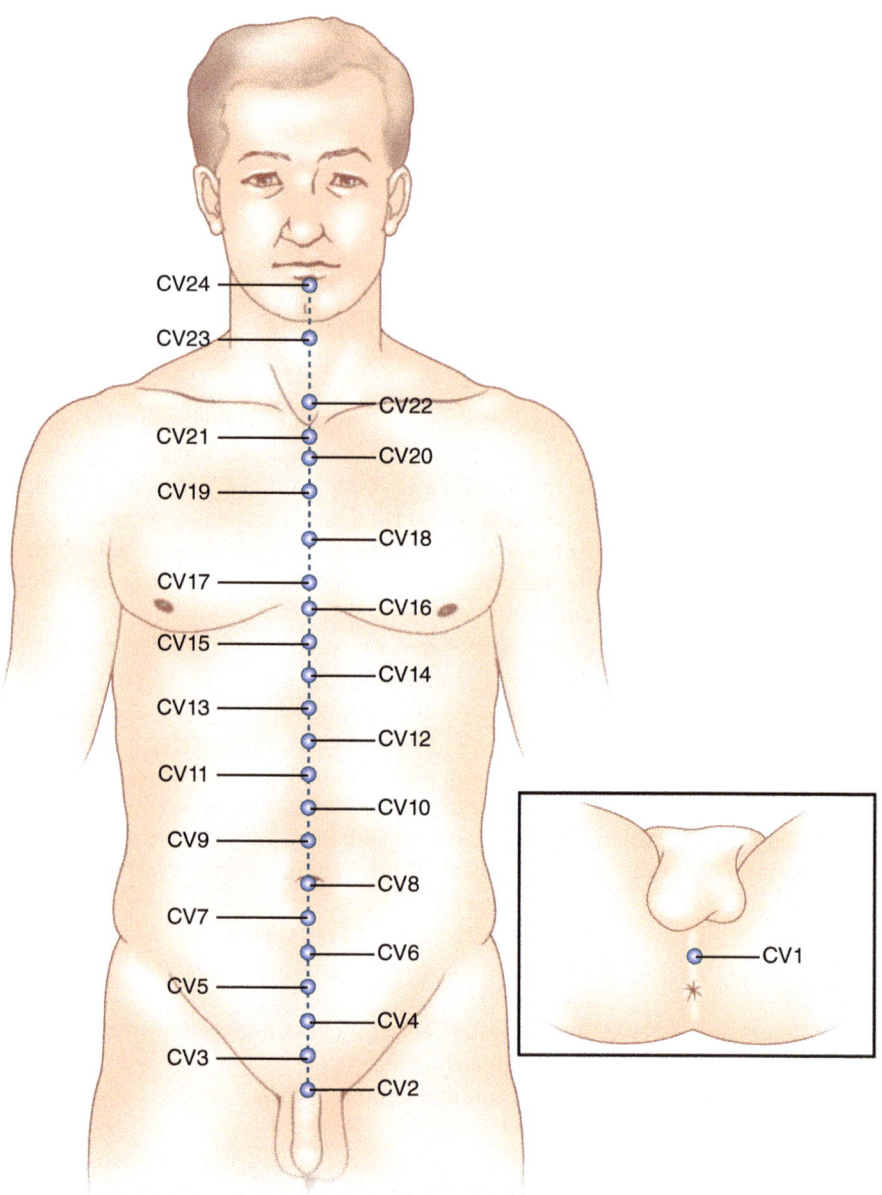

Fig. 22.1 Conception vessel

22 Conception Vessel 任脈經穴

CV 19 Zigong 紫宮	At the midline anterior chest, at the level of second intercostals.
CV 20 Huagai 華蓋	At the midline anterior chest, at the level of first intercostals.
CV 21 Xuanji 旋璣	At the anterior top midline of chest 0.5 tsun below the suprasternal notch.
CV 22 Tiantu 天突	At the anterior top midline of chest over the suprasternal notch.
CV 23 Lianquan 廉泉	At the anterior midline of neck over the front top notch of cricoids cartilage.
CV 24 Chengjiang 承漿	At the anterior midline, in the depression over the center of mentolabial groove (see Fig. 22.1).

Chapter 23
Governor Vessel 督脈經穴

Yuan-Chi Lin and Lynn M. Rusy

GV 1 Changgqian 長強	Midway between the anus and the coccyx.
GV 2 Yaoshu 腰俞	Midline at sacral hiatus.
GV 3 Yaoyangguan 腰陽關	In the depression inferior to the spinous process of fourth lumbar vertebrae.
GV 4 Mingmen 命門	In the depression inferior to the spinous process of second lumbar vertebrae.
GV 5 Xuanshu 懸樞	In the depression inferior to the spinous process of first lumbar vertebrae.
GV 6 Jizhong 脊中	In the depression inferior to the spinous process of eleventh thoracic vertebrae.
GV 7 Zhongshu 中樞	In the depression inferior to the spinous process of tenth thoracic vertebrae.
GV 8 Jinsuo 筋縮	In the depression inferior to the spinous process of ninth thoracic vertebrae.
GV 9 Zhiyang 至陽	In the depression inferior to the spinous process of seventh thoracic vertebrae.
GV 10 Lingtai 靈臺	In the depression inferior to the spinous process of sixth thoracic vertebrae.
GV 11 Shendao 神道	In the depression inferior to the spinous process of fifth thoracic vertebrae.
GV 12 Shenzhu 身柱	In the depression inferior to the spinous process of third thoracic vertebrae.
GV 13 Taodao 陶道	In the depression inferior to the spinous process of first thoracic vertebrae.

Y.-C. Lin (✉)
Medical Acupuncture Service, Department of Anesthesiology, Perioperative and Pain Medicine, Boston Children's Hospital, 300 Longwood Ave., Boston, Massachusetts 02115, USA

Department of Anaesthesia, Harvard Medical School, Boston, Massachusetts, USA
e-mail: yuan-chi.lin@childrens.harvard.edu

L. M. Rusy
Department of Anesthesia, Children's Hospital of Wisconsin, Milwaukee, Wisconsin, USA

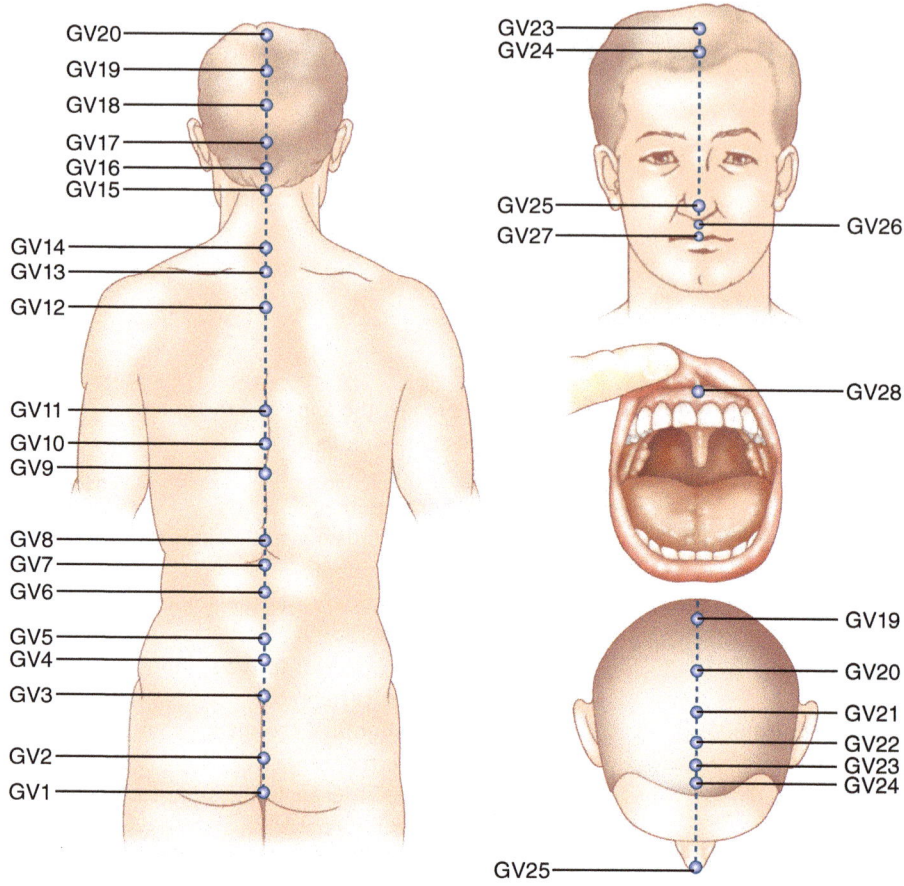

Fig. 23.1 Governor vessel

GV 14 DaiZhui 大椎	In the depression inferior to the spinous process of seventh cervical vertebrae.
GV 15 Yamen 啞門	In the depression inferior to the spinous process of second cervical vertebrae.
GV 16 Fengfu 風府	Directly inferior to the external occipital protuberance, in the depression of between trapezius muscles.
GV 17 Naohu 腦户	In the middepression superior to the external occipital protuberance.
GV 18 Qiangjian 强間	On the midline of posterior occiput, 1.5 tsun above the GV 17.
GV 19 Houdins 後頂	On the midline of posterior occiput, 1.5 tsun above the GV 18.

23 Governor Vessel 督脈經穴

GV 20 Baihui 百會	On the vertex of midsaggital line, at the midpoint of a line connecting the top of ear apexes.
GV 21 Q1anding 前頂	On the midsaggital line, 1.5 tsun anterior to the GV 20.
GV 22 Xinhui 顖會	On the midsaggital line, 3 tsun anterior to the GV 20.
GV 23 Shangxing 上星	On the midline above forehead, 4 tsun anterior to the GV 20.
GV 24 Shenting 神庭	On the midline forehead, 1/2 tsun within anterior hairline.
GV 25 Suliao 素髎	At the tip of nose.
GV 26 Shuigou 水溝	At the midline midpoint of philtrum.
GV 27 DuiDuan 兌端	At the midtip of upper lip tubercle.
GV 28 Yinjiao 齦交	At the midpoint between the upper lip and upper labial gingiva (See Fig. 23.1).

Chapter 24
The Extra Acupuncture Points 奇穴

Yuan-Chi Lin and Cynthia S. Tung

EX-HN1 Si Shen Chong 四神聰	Four points over the top of head, 1 tsun in the front, back, and bilateral of GV 20 (see Fig. 24.1).
EX-HN3 Yintang 印堂	Midway between the eyebrows (see Fig. 24.2).
EX-HN4 Yuyao 魚腰	In the midpoint of eyebrows above the eyeball when eyes are looking straight (see Fig. 24.3).
EX-HN5 Taiyang 太陽	In a depression, 1 tsun posterior to the midpoint between the lateral angle of eye and lateral end of eyebrow (see Fig. 24.4).
EX-HN6 Erjian 耳尖	On the tip of each ear (see Fig. 24.5).
Ex-HN7 Qiuhou 球後	Over the lower eyelid between outer one fourth and inner three fourth (see Fig. 24.6).
HuaTao Jai Ji 華佗夾脊	Half tsun lateral to the lower border of the spinal processes of vertebrae T1 to L5 with total of 34 points (see Fig. 24.7).
Yao Tong Dian 腰痛點	Two points on the dorsal side of hand: one in the depression near the base between the second and third metacarpal bones and the other between fourth and fifth metacarpal bones (see Fig. 24.8).
Ba Xie 八邪	Four points on each hand, over the dorsum of each hand proximal to the end of interdigital folds (see Fig. 24.9).
Ba Fen 八風	Four points on each foot, over the dorsum of each foot proximal to thsecond interphalangeal transverse foldse end of interdigital folds (see Fig. 24.10).

Y.-C. Lin (✉) · C. S. Tung
Medical Acupuncture Service, Department of Anesthesiology, Perioperative and Pain Medicine, Boston Children's Hospital, 300 Longwood Ave., Boston, Massachusetts 02115, USA

Department of Anaesthesia, Harvard Medical School, Boston, Massachusetts, USA
e-mail: yuan-chi.lin@childrens.harvard.edu

Fig. 24.1 Si Shen Chong

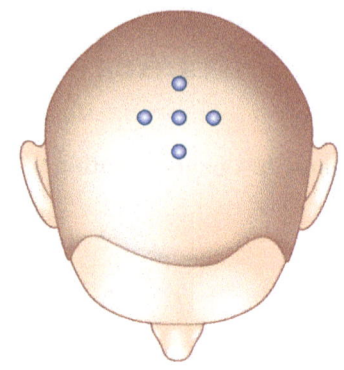

Fig. 24.2 Yintang

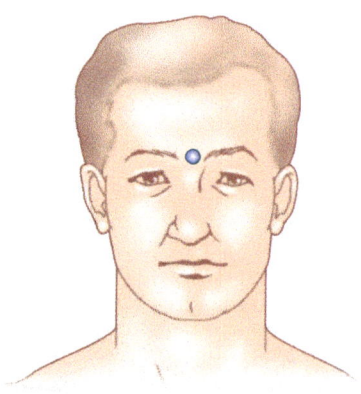

Fig. 24.3 Yuyao

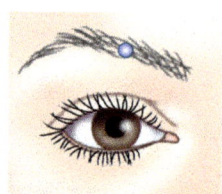

24 The Extra Acupuncture Points 奇穴

Fig. 24.4 Taiyang

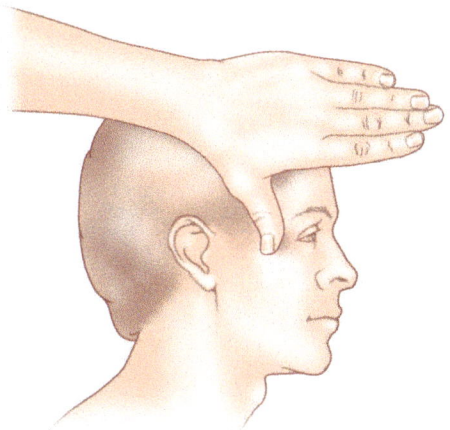

Fig. 24.5 Erjian

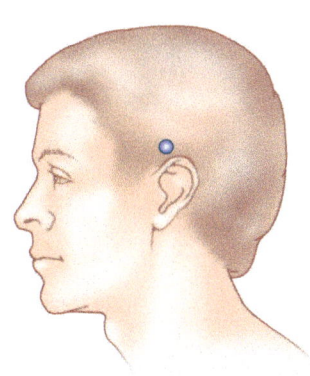

Fig. 24.6 Qiuhou

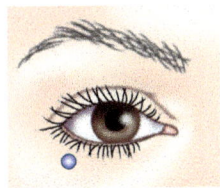

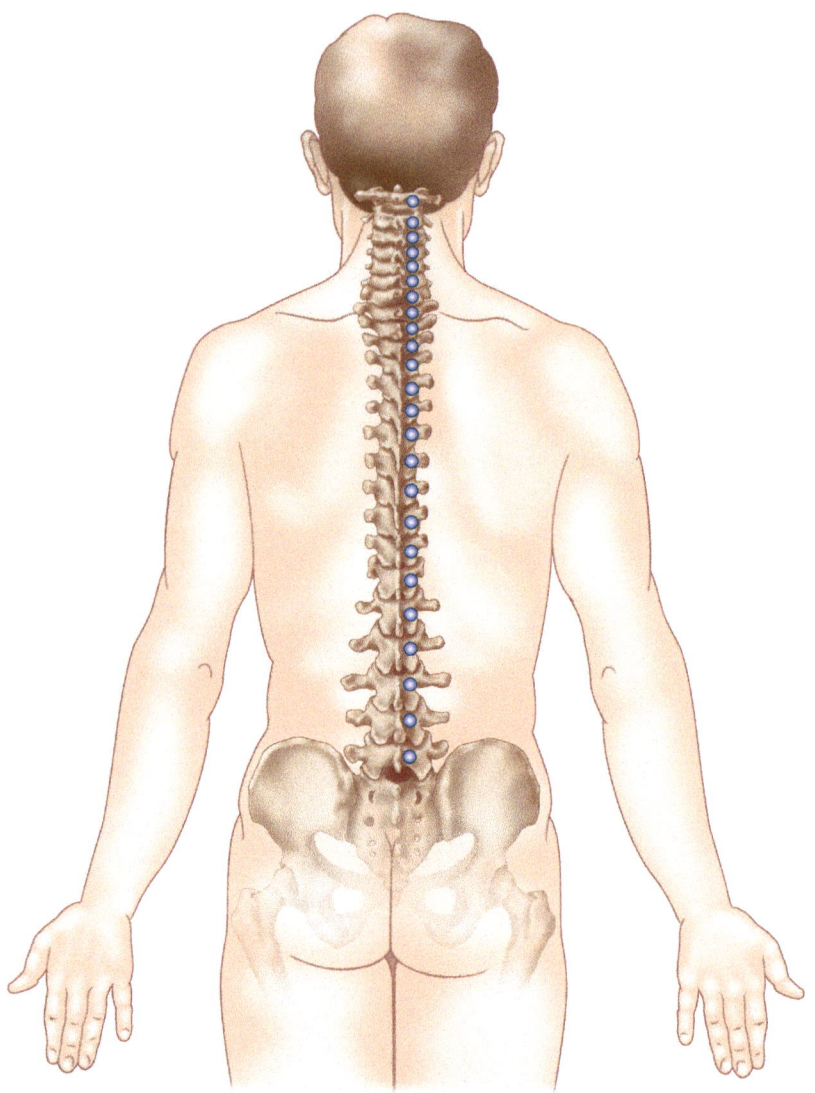

Fig. 24.7 HuaTao Jai Ji

24 The Extra Acupuncture Points 奇穴

Fig. 24.8 Yao Tung Dian

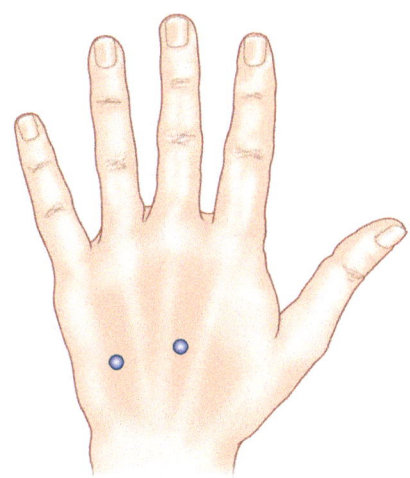

Fig. 24.9 Ba Xie

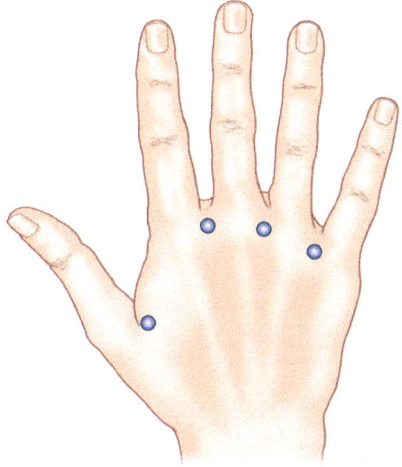

Fig. 24.10 Ba Fen

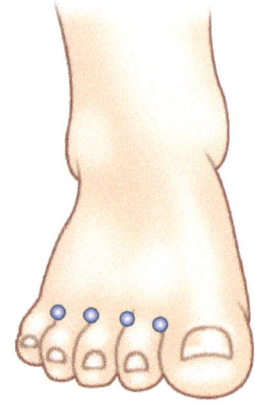

Fig. 24.11 Si Feng

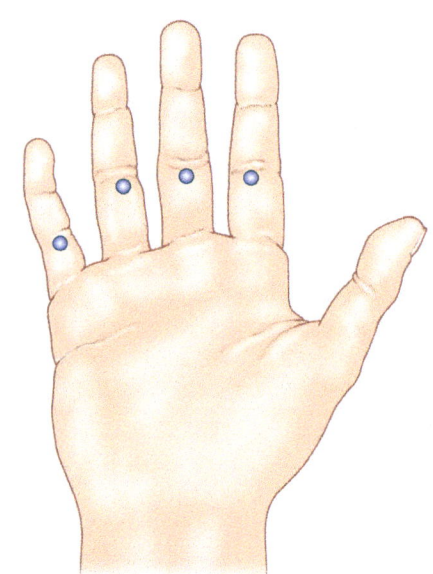

Fig. 24.12 Qi Yen

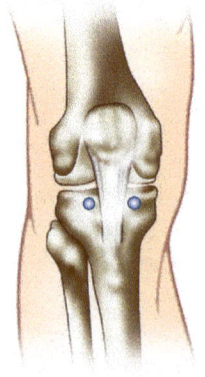

24 The Extra Acupuncture Points 奇穴

Si Feng 四縫	Except the thumbs, over the ventral side of hand, between the first and second interphalangeal transverse folds (see Fig. 24.11).
Qi Yen 膝眼	In the depressions on both sides below patella. Lateral Qi Yen is also ST 35 acupuncture point (see Fig. 24.12).
Asi Points 阿是穴	Tenderness acupuncture points.

Part III
Clinical Conditions

Chapter 25
Headache

Jaung-Geng Lin, Kuen-Bao Chen and Yu-Chen Lee

Cause and Mechanism of Disease

In modern medicine, there are different diagnostic criteria for headache, generally divided into migraine, cluster headache, and tension headache.

Migraine

In patients with migraine headache, the location of the pain is usually unilateral or bilateral at the temple or forehead, and is more common in females than males. Migraine headaches are pulsating in nature, and are often accompanied by nausea and vomiting. There may be precursor symptoms present before onset of the headache, such as sparking and flashing before eyes, sensitivity to light, blind spots, dizziness, and tinnitus. These headaches usually occur when a patient wakes up in the morning or in the evening, and may last from several hours to 1–2 days. The period is irregular, which ranges from several weeks to several months. Onset of migraine headache is less common at noontime, and during pregnancy, the symptoms will often lessen or disappear. Some factors, such as glare, noise, and consumption of alcohol, may increase the intensity of headache. Sleep and local compression often reduces these symptoms.

K.-B. Chen (✉)
Department of Anesthesiology, China Medical University Hospital,
2 Yuh-Der Road, North District, Taichung, Taiwan 40447, Republic of China
e-mail: d3510@mail.cmuh.org.tw
e-mail: kpc329@yahoo.com.tw

J.-G. Lin
School of Chinese Medicine, China Medical University, Taichung,
Taiwan, Republic of China

Y.-C. Lee
Department of Acupuncture, China Medical University Hospital,
Taichung, Taiwan, Republic of China

Cluster Headache

Cluster headaches are located unilaterally at the orbit or temple, and occur most frequently in adolescent and adult males. The pain is severe but nonpulsating in nature, and is accompanied by tears and congestion of the eyes. Cluster headaches usually occur at night, typically one to several hours after onset of sleep. These headaches rarely occur during the day, and the most common trigger is alcohol.

Tension Headache

Tension headaches are usually bilateral, starting in the neck and back and extending to the head and bilateral forehead, although local pain is also common. The headache is oppressive and tension filled in nature, rather than pulsating. The onset is continuous and repetitive, and the intensity may vary, lasting from several hours to several days, or even months. Patients typically present with characteristics such as nervousness, anxiety and insomnia, and these headaches are more likely to occur when the patient is tired or nervous.

Some headaches are a result of organic changes in the body, such as head trauma, meningitis, brain tumor, and temporal arteritis. It is important to examine the patient and treat with modern medicine to establish the diagnosis.

Treatment

Body Acupuncture

When treating headaches with acupuncture, choose acupoints along the meridian of the major headache region. The main acupoints for treatment of headache are GB 20 (Fengchi), GV 20 (Baihui), EX-HN5 (Taiyang), LI 4 (Hegu), LU 7 (Lieque), and SI 3 (Houxi). If forehead pain is located at the frontal region of the head, which is passed through by the bladder meridian, the governor vessel meridian, and the gallbladder meridian, add acupoints such as GV 23 (Shangxing), GB 14 (Yangbai), EX-HN3 (Yintang), and BL 2 (Cuanzhu). If a migraine headache is located at the lateral head region, add acupoints such as GB 8 (Shuaigu), TE 5 (Waiguan), ST 8 (Touwei), and GB 40 (Qiuxu). If the headache is located at the occipital region passed through by the bladder meridian and the governor vessel meridian, add BL 10 (Tianzhu), GV 14 (Dazhui), and BL 11 (Dazhu). For pain at the top of the head, add EX-HN1 (Si Shen Chong) and LR 3 (Taichong). For wind-heat headache, add GV 14 (Dazhui) and LI 11 (Quchi).

Ear Acupuncture

When using ear acupuncture to treat headache, one may use AT 3 (Zhen; occiput), AT 1 (E; forehead), AT 2 (Nie; temple), MA-AT (Naodian; brain), TF 4 (Shenmen), and CO 12 (Gan; liver). The most effective treatment takes 3–4 acupoints per session with strong stimulation, needle retention for 20–30 min, and twisting every 5 min. One may also use buried needle method or pasted beans method, and teach the patients to push the needle themselves.

Chapter 26
Facial Nerve Palsy

Jaung-Geng Lin, Kuen-Bao Chen and Yu-Chen Lee

Treatment

Acupuncture at the meridian of Hand-Yangming and Foot-Yangming, supplemented with meridian of Foot-Taiyang, is the primary treatment for facial nerve palsy. Draining method is used in the primary stage of external contraction, with meridian physiotherapy or tonifying method with moxibustion used in the later stage. The main acupuncture points for facial nerve palsy treatment are GB 20 (Fengchi), GB 14 (Yangbai), BL 2 (Cuanzhu), LI 20 (Yingxiang), ST 4 (Dicang), ST 6 (Jiache), SJ 17 (Yifung), and LI 4 (Hegu). Acupuncture points Dicang-penetrating-Jiache, Jiache-penetrating-Chuanliao, Taiyang-penetrating-Jiache, SJ 17 (Yifung), SJ 21 (Ermen), GB 14 (Yangbai), ST 8 (Touwei), GV 23 (Shangxing), EX-HN3 (Yintang), LI 20 (Yingxiang), ipsilateral LI 4(Hegu), bilateral ST 36 (Zusanli), and LR 3 (Taichong) are also effective as assist points, which can be used by turns with good results to treat periphery-type facial nerve palsy.

K.-B. Chen (✉)
Department of Anesthesiology, China Medical University Hospital,
2 Yuh-Der Road, North District, Taichung, Taiwan 40447, Republic of China
e-mail: d3510@mail.cmuh.org.tw
e-mail: kpc329@yahoo.com.tw

J.-G. Lin
School of Chinese Medicine, China Medical University,
Taichung, Taiwan, Republic of China

Y.-C. Lee
Department of Acupuncture, China Medical University Hospital,
Taichung, Taiwan, Republic of China

Notes

In cases of facial nerve palsy after infection or trauma, if the condition has not improved after receiving acupuncture treatment for a period of more than 1 month, further examination is required to exclude organic lesions (such as tumor) and avoid prolonging the illness. In acute onset of facial nerve palsy, it is inappropriate to perform electroacupuncture or electrotherapy on local affected area. If the patient feels heat or pain at local affected area, hot compresses, massage, or chewing gum should not be advised, as it is important to avoid stirring wind and wind-heat diffusion.

Chapter 27
Vertigo

Jaung-Geng Lin, Kuen-Bao Chen and Yu-Chen Lee

Overview

Vertigo is feeling dizzy, seeing things rotating and overturning, and an inability to sit or stand. It is often accompanied by symptoms like nausea, vomiting, and sweating. In mild cases, these symptoms will cease when the eyes are closed, and will relieve in time. In severe cases, the patient may feel as if he or she is on a boat or in a car, or that the world keeps rotating. They may be unable to stand up or may even faint. The symptoms of vertigo are sometimes found in patients with high blood pressure, arteriosclerosis, inner ear vertigo, anemia, and neurasthenia.

Syndrome Differentiation and Treatment

Clinical Manifestation

Deficiency Syndrome Dizziness without the sensation of rotating or seeing things overturn is a common symptom. Symptoms reoccur and worsen with fatigue. The patient is blanched and appears tired, and may experience palpitations, sleep loss, backache, tinnitus, pale tongue body, and weak pulse.

K.-B. Chen (✉)
Department of Anesthesiology, China Medical University Hospital,
2 Yuh-Der Road, North District, Taichung, Taiwan 40447, Republic of China
e-mail: d3510@mail.cmuh.org.tw
e-mail: kpc329@yahoo.com.tw

J.-G. Lin
School of Chinese Medicine, China Medical University,
Taichung, Taiwan, Republic of China

Y.-C. Lee
Department of Acupuncture, China Medical University Hospital,
Taichung, Taiwan, Republic of China

Excess Syndrome Vertigo is paroxysmal. The patient sees things rotating and overturning, suffers from headache or giddiness, is fidgety or angry, and experiences swelling of the chest and hypochondrium, nausea, and vomiting. Appetite is poor, and the patient has reddish tongue body with a thick or yellow coating on it. The pulse is contracture or smooth.

Treatment

Deficiency Syndrome

Treatment Nourish qi and blood. Select the transport point, governor vessel, and meridian points including Zu Shao Yang and Yang Ming. Tonifying method is appropriate for the needle and moxibustion is allowed.

Prescription The prescribed points are GV 20 (Baihui), GB 20 (Fengchi), BL 18 (Ganshu), BL 23 (Shenshu), and ST 36 (Zusanli).

Method (Fang yi) GV 20 (Baihui) moxibustion elevates Qing Yang, GB 20 (Fengchi) moxibustion eliminates internal wind, BL 18 (Ganshu) and BL 23 (Shenshu) are effective for blood nourishing and essence production, BL 20 (Pishu) and ST 36 (Zusanli) are for center nourishing and beneficial for qi. Original qi, essence, is enriched, as is the blood, and the sea of marrow is nourished, relieving the vertigo.

Acupuncture Point Selection with additional symptoms Add PC 6 (Neiguan) when palpitation is present; add HT 7 (Shenmen) for sleep loss; and add SI 19 (Tingkung) for tinnitus.

Excess Syndrome

Treatment Pacify the liver to subdue yang and harmonize the stomach to resolve phlegm. Select conception vessel, governor vessel, and Three Ying meridian of the foot. Draining method is appropriate for the needle, and moxibustion is not allowed.

Prescription The prescribed points are CV 12 (Chungwan), SP 9 (Yinlingquan), LR 2 (Xingjian), KI 5 (Shuichuan), and Ex-Hn3 (Yintang).

Method (Fang yi) "All winds diaoxuan belong to liver." LR 2 (Xingjian) is selected to pacify the liver and downbear counterflow, KI 5 (Shuichuan) nourishes yin and subdues yang, Yintang is an extra point, which is good for head and eye clearing and for relieving vertigo. Stomach mu CV 12 (Chungwan) is also selected to harmonize center and ease vomiting. Spleen connected with SP 9 (Yinlingquan) fortifies the spleen to resolve dampness, which resolves phlegm. If there is no phlegm, there will be no vertigo. For a vertigo patient presenting with liver yang with phlegm turbidity ascending counterflow, this recipe is more appropriate.

Acupuncture Point Selection with Additional Symptoms Add SP 9 (Yinlingquan) when distention is present and add ST 8 (Touwei) when the head is heavy.

Chapter 28
Toothache

Jaung-Geng Lin, Kuen-Bao Chen and Yu-Chen Lee

Treatment

The main acupuncture points for treatment of toothache are LI 4 (Hegu), ST 44 (Neiting), ST 6 (Jiache), GB 2 (Tinghui), and LI 11 (Quchi). Meridian of Hand-Yangming Hegu is the most effective acupuncture point for toothache treatment. During treatment, first acupuncture Hegulateral to the pain. Insert the needle at an upper oblique angle until patient feels an electric-like tingle in the arm, then use a bird pecking operation until the pain stops and withdraw the needle. If the pain cannot be stopped, acupuncture Hegu of another hand. If the pain still cannot be stopped, acupuncture ST 44 (Neiting), ST 4 (Dicang), ST 6 (Jiache), and SJ 21 (Ermen) until the pain stops.

Characteristic Explanation

LI 4 (Hegu) belongs to the meridian of Hand-Yangming, and Neiting belongs to stomach meridian of Foot-Yangming. The meridians of both Hand-Yangming and Foot-Yangming pass through alveolus, so using needles to prick Hegu and Neiting can treat toothache pain. However, deficient fire fluctuation caused by kidney deficiency and liver fire is still common, so acupuncture points such as KI 3 (Taixi) and LR 3 (Taichong) should also be considered.

Notes

Toothache caused by lack of sleep, gum inflammation, gum prominence, and chewing difficulties caused by fire heat can all be treated by acupuncture in conjunction with drugs. In cases of acute pulpitis, it is necessary to refer the patient to a dentist.

Chapter 29
Neck Pain

Jaung-Geng Lin, Kuen-Bao Chen and Yu-Chen Lee

Treatment

The main treatment acupuncture points for neck pain are GB 20 (Fengchi), GV 14 (Daizhui), GB 21 (Jianjing), SI 9 (Jianzhen), SJ 5 (Waiguan), GB 39 (Xuanzhong), KI 3 (Houxi), and Tienying acupuncture points (Ahshi acupuncture point). If Foot-Taiyang meridian is sick, then add BL 10 (Tianzhu), DU 14 (Dazhu), and BL 60 (Kunlun) acupuncture points. If lesser yang meridian is sick, add SJ 17 (Yifeng), SJ 5 (Waiguan), and GB 34 (Yanglingquan) acupuncture points. Pick neck sprain points for hand needles. Use plum blossom needle from periphery to nidus and prick successively according to muscle and meridian parts. The technique should start light at first, then become heavy until local skin redness or a small amount of bleeding occurs. During the operation, tell the patient to move his or her neck. This is a stirring qi therapy.

Chapter 30
Chest Pain

Jaung-Geng Lin, Kuen-Bao Chen and Yu-Chen Lee

Treatment

Mainly use PC 6 (Neiguan), LU 5 (Chize), RN 17 (Danzhong), and BL 15 (Xinshu) for treatment of chest pain. For stabbing chest pain, which is fixed and without movement, add BL 14 (Jueyinshu), BI 17 (Geshu), and LR 3 (Taichong). For chest tightness with pain, or pain throughout chest and back, add BL 13 (Feishu), ST 40 (Fenglong), and RN 12 (Zhongwan). For weakness with chest pain throughout the back, which will be more severe when it is cold, add BL 14 (Jueyingshu) and PC 4 (Ximen).

Chapter 31
Epigastric Pain

Jaung-Geng Lin, Kuen-Bao Chen and Yu-Chen Lee

Treatment

The main acupuncture points for treatment of epigastric pain are ST 44 (Neiting), ST 36 (Zusanli), PC 6 (Neiguan), CV 13 (Shangwan), BL 20 (Pishu), SP 4 (Gongsun), BL 17 (Geshu), and BL 21 (Weishu). Clinical investigation demonstrates that chronic atrophic gastritis treated with acupuncture points such as T 7–T 12 Huatuojiaji and ST 36 (Zusanli) achieves good results.

Notes

For epigastric pain treatment, acupuncture PC 6 (Neiguan) and ST 36 (Zusanli) first and then acupuncture the upper, medium, and lower three stomachs (Renmai, the acupuncture point that is at the surface near stomach). Acupuncture with moxibustion can be used. Pishu and Weishu moxibustions can be added for chronic epigastric pain.

K.-B. Chen (✉)
Department of Anesthesiology, China Medical University Hospital,
2 Yuh-Der Road, North District, Taichung, Taiwan 40447, Republic of China
e-mail: d3510@mail.cmuh.org.tw
e-mail: kpc329@yahoo.com.tw

J.-G. Lin
School of Chinese Medicine, China Medical University,
Taichung, Taiwan, Republic of China

Y.-C. Lee
Department of Acupuncture, China Medical University Hospital,
Taichung, Taiwan, Republic of China

Concerning acupuncture for stomach pain treatment, moxibustion can also be used. Stomach pain patients should be careful about their diet and must be particularly vigilant about their breakfasts. In addition, it is beneficial for them to maintain spirit relaxation, abstain from smoking, avoid alcohol and betel nuts, maintain a healthy diet, and consume smaller meals at more frequent intervals to reduce their rate of relapse and promote recovery.

Chapter 32
Abdominal Pain

Jaung-Geng Lin, Kuen-Bao Chen and Yu-Chen Lee

Abdominal pain is characterized primarily by pain in the abdominal region neighboring the umbilicus. It is commonly seen in patients with gastritis, duodenitis, gastric ulcer, and duodenal ulcers.

Treatment

The main points to treat abdominal pain are ST 44 (Neiting), ST 36 (Zhusanli), PC 6 (Neiguan), CV 12 (Zhongwan), BL 20 (Pishu), SP 4 (Gongsun), BL 17 (Geshu), BL 21 (Weishu), etc. According to clinical research, excellent results can be obtained by treating chronic atrophic gastritis (CAG) by needling Ex-B-2 (Jia-Ji points) from T 7 to T 12 and ST 36 (Zhusanli).

ST 36 (Zhusanli) is a point from the stomach meridian, which can be combined with PC 6 (Neiguan) and SP 4 (Gongsun) as Eight Confluential Points to treat pain in the heart, chest, and epigastric area. CV 12 (Zhongwan) is the Front-Mu Point of stomach, which is located in the middle of stomach. It is the main point for treating abdominal pain by needling or moxibustion.

K.-B. Chen (✉)
Department of Anesthesiology, China Medical University Hospital,
2 Yuh-Der Road, North District, Taichung, Taiwan 40447, Republic of China
e-mail: d3510@mail.cmuh.org.tw
e-mail: kpc329@yahoo.com.tw

J.-G. Lin
School of Chinese Medicine, China Medical University,
Taichung, Taiwan, Republic of China

Y.-C. Lee
Department of Acupuncture, China Medical University Hospital,
Taichung, Taiwan, Republic of China

Caution

1. To treat abdominal pain, one should start from PC 6 (Neiguan) and ST 36 (Zhusanli) and then needle CV 13 (Shangwan), CV 12 (Zhongwan), and CV 10 (Xiawan). Warming needle can be done on those points. One can also perform moxibustion at BL 20 (Pishu) and BL 21 (Weishu) for chronic abdominal pain.
2. Moxibustion can be combined with needling when treating epigastric pain.
3. Patients with abdominal pain should pay close attention to their diet, taking particular care to eat breakfast and maintain a relaxed mood. To prevent relapse and achieve recovery, one should avoid smoking and chewing betel nuts and eat smaller, more frequent regular meals.

Chapter 33
Dysmenorrhea

Jaung-Geng Lin, Kuen-Bao Chen and Yu-Chen Lee

Etiology and Pathology

Dysmenorrhea is lower abdominal pain or pain radiating to lumbosacral region before, during, or after menstruation. Primary dysmenorrhea, also known as functional dysmenorrheal, refers to pain without organic pathological changes to the reproductive organs. Menstrual pain due to pathological changes in the reproductive organs is called secondary dysmenorrhea, which may occur in patients with endometriosis, pelvic inflammation, and uterine myoma.

The main symptoms of primary dysmenorrhea are intermittent colic, distention pain or pain with a falling sensation in the lower abdomen, or pain radiating to lumbosacral region, which is a severe pain radiating to medial side of thigh, vagina, and anus. Most patients experience cramping in the lower abdomen and increased menstrual flow and note a preference for pressure and warmth, which helps alleviate the pain.

In some cases, dysmenorrhea may be accompanied by digestive symptoms, such as nausea, vomiting, and diarrhea. Patients may also present with frequent urination, urgent urination, distending and falling sensations of the anus, pale complexion, profuse cold sweating, cold hands and feet, and syncope in severe cases.

K.-B. Chen (✉)
Department of Anesthesiology, China Medical University Hospital,
2 Yuh-Der Road, North District, Taichung, Taiwan 40447, Republic of China
e-mail: d3510@mail.cmuh.org.tw
e-mail: kpc329@yahoo.com.tw

J.-G. Lin
School of Chinese Medicine, China Medical University,
Taichung, Taiwan, Republic of China

Y.-C. Lee
Department of Acupuncture, China Medical University Hospital,
Taichung, Taiwan, Republic of China

Treatment

Body Acupuncture

The main points to treat dysmenorrhea are BL 31–BL 34 (Baliaoxue is Shangliao, Ciliao, Zhongliao, Xialiao), SP 4 (Gongsun), SP 6 (Sanyinjiao), GB 34 (Yanglingquan), LIV 3 (Taichong), KID 3 (Taixi), SP 10 (Xuehai), ST 25 (Tianshu), PC 6 (Neiguan), LI 4 (Hegu), Zi-Gong (Ex-CA-1), etc.

Ear Acupuncture/Auricular Points

In treating dysmenorrhea with ear acupuncture, one can select uterus, endocrine, sympathetic, ear Shen Men, ovary, and kidney. At each treatment, one may needle 2–4 points with mild stimulation, retaining the needles for 20 min, once per day. In severe cases, use cutaneous needling method and have the patients press the needling area to strengthen stimulation during the treatment period.

Moxibustion Therapy

To treat dysmenorrhea, one may use moxa on CV 4 (Guanyuan), CV 3 (Zhongji), CV 6 (Qihai), SP 6 (Sanyinjiao), etc. The method is done by using the moxa to warm these points 2–3 days before the period or during the period for 15–20 min, once or twice per day. If the patient suffers from near-collapse due to severe dysmenorrhea accompanied by menorrhagia, one can use moxa on GV 20 (Baihui) or CV 4 (Guanyuan). This method can also be used to treat patients with syncope due to excess hemorrhage.

If the patient does not experience heavy bleeding, 3–5 cones of ginger moxa can be used on CV 8 (Shenque), SP 1 (Yingbai), and GV 3 (Yaoyangguan).

According to clinical research, excellent results can be obtained in the treatment of primary dysmenorrhea by needling SP 6 (Sanyinjiao) and moxibustion at CV 4 (Guanyuan), CV 6 (Qihai), and BL 23 (Shenshu).

Caution

Acupuncture has a pronounced effect on alleviating pain in primary dysmenorrhea. Acupuncture and moxibustion can be helpful in relieving symptoms of secondary dysmenorrhea caused by endometriosis, pelvic inflammation, and uterine myoma. It is best to treat dysmenorrhea with acupuncture starting 3–5 days before menstruation and continuing until the end of the period. Patient should receive treatments for three consecutive menstrual cycles. They should avoid raw and cold foods and emphasis should be placed on exercise.

Chapter 34
Upper Back Pain

Jaung-Geng Lin, Kuen-Bao Chen and Yu-Chen Lee

Common Causes of Upper Back Pain

Upper back pain is often caused by improper posture, which overstrains the muscles of upper back (including the trapezius muscle, rhomboid major and minor muscle, splenius cervicis muscle, longissimus thoracis muscle, iliocostalis thoracis muscle, etc.). Imbalanced distribution of force exerted on the upper back muscles due to scoliosis may also cause upper back pain, as may sprained muscles, ankylosing spondylitis (AS), senile kyphosis, and rheumatic arthritis (RA).

Treatment

The main acupuncture points for treatment of upper back pain are GB 21 (Jianjing), BL 11 (Dazhu), GV 14 (Daizhui), BL 12 (Fengmen), BL 13 (Feishu), BL 14 (Jueyinshu), BL 15 (Xinshu), BL 17 (Geshu), SI 11 (Tianzong), SI 12 (Bingfeng), SI 13 (Quyuan), and SI 3 (Houxi), etc. Acupuncture or moxibustion can also be used, according to syndrome differentiation. EX-B-2 (Hua Tuo Jia-Ji points) may also be selected, and cupping the painful area may be used as well.

The main acupuncture prescription to treat upper back pain is selected acupuncture points from bladder meridian, small intestine meridian, and governing vessel, as well as distal points to manipulate with Moving-Qi-Therapy. The treatment can also be combined with moxibustion and cupping to relax muscle tension and alleviate pain.

Caution

Avoid carrying heavy, oversized objects with slippery surfaces and use tools that reduce the mechanical burden on the upper back. Adopt proper posture, stand with a straight back with the jaw retracted and neck straight. Stick out the chest, pull back the abdomen, and balance both shoulders. Putting each leg up on a stool in an alternating manner can reduce pressure on the upper back for those that have to stand for long periods of time.

Chapter 35
Frozen Shoulder

Jaung-Geng Lin, Kuen-Bao Chen and Yu-Chen Lee

Etiology and Pathology

Frozen shoulder is a condition that occurs primarily in middle-aged individuals. The clinical signs of frozen shoulder include shoulder pain, which may occur gradually, sometimes manifesting as a cutting or dull pain and may radiate toward front shoulder and scapula area. Severe shoulder pain may cause pronounced sleep disturbance.

Patients with shoulder pain may experience difficulty combing their hair or dressing due to limited abduction, external rotation, and elevation of the shoulder joint. Some patients may have multiple points of tenderness, whereas others are tender in a more local area. Some suffer from muscular atrophy as well, particularly in the deltoid muscle. The course of disease in most cases is generally months and even years in some cases.

Major Points for Diagnosis

The onset of frozen shoulder is soreness, which starts on one or both sides, and may radiate to neck and whole upper limb. The pain worsens at night. The affected shoulder may display an aversion to wind-cold and the fingers may become

---

K.-B. Chen (✉)
Department of Anesthesiology, China Medical University Hospital,
2 Yuh-Der Road, North District, Taichung, Taiwan 40447, Republic of China
e-mail: d3510@mail.cmuh.org.tw
e-mail: kpc329@yahoo.com.tw

J.-G. Lin
School of Chinese Medicine, China Medical University,
Taichung, Taiwan, Republic of China

Y.-C. Lee
Department of Acupuncture, China Medical University Hospital,
Taichung, Taiwan, Republic of China

numb and distended. The shoulder joint may show varying levels of stiffness and the abduction, external rotation, and elevation of shoulder joint become limited.

Treatment

Treating the pain is the major goal at the initial stage, with improving the impaired function as the primary goal in the late stage. The main acupuncture points to treat frozen shoulder are LI 15 (Jianyu), TE 14 (Jianliao), SI 9 (Jianzhen), LI 14 (Binao), SI 11 (Tianzong), LI 16 (Jugu), LI 11 (Quchi), LI 4 (Hegu), and Ah-Shi points. One can also add ST 38 (Tiaokou) penetrated to UB 57 (Chenshang), GB 34 (Yanglingquan), or manipulation with Moving-Qi-Therapy.

Caution

Patients can do rehabilitative exercises to alleviate pain:

1. Pendulum exercise: With the healthy shoulder resting on a table and the affected shoulder drooping down in a relaxed manner, shake the entire trunk in order to radiate a wave of movement to the shoulder joint and bring about flexion, extension, abduction, and adduction.
2. Climb the ladder exercise: Facing forward or sideways to the wall, lift shoulder on lateral side and move fingers up and down as if climbing a ladder.
3. Shrugging shoulder exercise: Move shoulder joint up and down, forward and back, and rotate internally and externally.

Chapter 36
Low Back Pain

Jaung-Geng Lin, Kuen-Bao Chen and Yu-Chen Lee

Among the diseases that lead to lower back pain, pathological lesion of the soft tissue is the most common, secondary to diseases of joints. Fewer incidences of lower back pain are the result of vascular pathology. Overstrain injuries are most commonly encountered in soft tissue pathology.

1. Acute lumbar sprain: Most commonly caused by indirect external force from improper bending postures and exertion of force
2. Chronic lumbar strain: Usually caused by prolonged bending, improper postures, and congenital malformations
3. Integrated facet syndrome: Often due to injury and subluxation of facet joints during exercise or weight-bearing activities
4. Injury of interspinous and supraspinous ligaments: Occurs with twisting motions or sudden changes of posture
5. Integrated lumbar transverse process syndrome: Usually caused by tension or muscle spasm at the waist and back due to labor or attack of wind-cold
6. Sprain injury of joints and partial dislocation (semiluxation): Caused by imbalance of force on the muscles from improper posture
7. Damage of superior cluneal nerves: Caused by sudden rotation to the right and left side
8. Piriformis muscle syndrome: Caused by overstrain of piriformis muscle
9. Sciatica: Caused by interstitial neuritis or compression of sciatic nerve

---

K.-B. Chen (✉)
Department of Anesthesiology, China Medical University Hospital,
2 Yuh-Der Road, North District, Taichung, Taiwan 40447, Republic of China
e-mail: d3510@mail.cmuh.org.tw
e-mail: kpc329@yahoo.com.tw

J.-G. Lin
School of Chinese Medicine, China Medical University,
Taichung, Taiwan, Republic of China

Y.-C. Lee
Department of Acupuncture, China Medical University Hospital,
Taichung, Taiwan, Republic of China

10. Prolapse of lumbar intervertebral disc: With increasing age, the lumbar intervertebral disc may degenerate, show atrophy, and show a decrease in elasticity, which can lead to protrusion of intervertebral discs. According to statistics, about 90% of disc herniation takes place between L4 and L5, and L5 and S1, which may bear the most stress of the body. Many cases occur between the age of 24 and 45 years

Treatment

The main points to treat lumbar pain are BL 23 (Shenshu), BL 52 (Zhishi), GV 3 (Yaoyangguan), BL 40 (Weizhong), SI 3 (Houxi), GB 39 (Xuanzhong), A-Shi points, and other trigger points. This prescription can be modified by the addition of GV 4 (Mingmen), SP 9 (Yinlingquan) for invasion of cold dampness, BL 17 (Geshu), GV 26 (Shuigou), BL 32 (Ciliao) for chronic strain, GV 4 (Mingmen), BL 52 (Zhishi), BL 58 (Feiyang), and KI 3 (Taixi) for kidney deficiency. According to clinical research, excellent results may be obtained by needling Ex-UE-7 (Yao-Tong-Dian*) when treating acute lumbar sprain. If the patient suffers from sudden onset of severe lumbar pain, one may prick and cup Ah-Shi points or use a three-edge needle to prick and induce bleeding at BL 40 (Weizhong).

Caution

1. Avoid long-term fixed postures or repetitive motion based on a single posture. For example, squatting after prolonged periods of standing can relax the muscles of waist and legs and reduce the consumption of energy.
2. Patient should pay attention to their posture when lifting heavy objects, squatting with the knees bent as they approach the object to avoid bending at the lower back and overloading it.
3. Obese patients should lose weight to reduce the burden to the lumbar region.

Chapter 37
Arthritis, Joint Pain

Jaung-Geng Lin, Kuen-Bao Chen and Yu-Chen Lee

The common arthritic diseases we see in clinic are rheumatoid arthritis, osteoarthritis, and gouty arthritis.

The Major Points for Diagnosis

The clinical signs of arthritis are soreness of the joints and soreness, heaviness, and numbness in parts of the muscles. When the condition persists, it may cause tightness and stiffness in the limbs, spasm, swelling, deformities of the joint, and so on. Patients may experience limited movement due to contracture deformity and sharp pain from flexing and extending.

Treatment

In consideration of the different types of pain and affected areas, one can select points from the local area, meridians, and syndrome differentiations as main points and add Ah-Shi points as supplementary points.

K.-B. Chen (✉)
Department of Anesthesiology, China Medical University Hospital,
2 Yuh-Der Road, North District, Taichung, Taiwan 40447, Republic of China
e-mail: d3510@mail.cmuh.org.tw
e-mail: kpc329@yahoo.com.tw

J.-G. Lin
School of Chinese Medicine, China Medical University,
Taichung, Taiwan, Republic of China

Y.-C. Lee
Department of Acupuncture, China Medical University Hospital,
Taichung, Taiwan, Republic of China

The treatment methods include shallow needling, cutaneous needle tapping, deep needling with long retention, moxa or warming needle, and cupping.

Following points should be selected from different affected areas to treat arthritis:

- Shoulder area: LI 15 (Jianyu), TE 14 (Jianliao), SI 10 (Naoshu), LI 4 (Hegu), TE 5 (Waiguan), SI 3 (Houxi)
- Elbow area: PC 3 (Quze), LU 5 (Chize), LI 11 (Quchi), TE 10 (Tianjing), TE 5 (Waiguan)
- Wrist area: PC 7 (Daling), TE 4 (Yangchi), TE 5 (Waiguan), LI 5 (Yangxi), SI 4 (Wangu)
- Finger Joints: LI 2 (Erjian), TE 3 (Zhongzhu), SI 2 (Qiangu), BaXie (EX-UE-9)
- Back spinal area: DU 26 (Shuigou), DU 12 (Shengzhu), DU 4 (Mingmen), DU 3 (Yaoyangguan)
- Knee area: Xi Yan (EX-LE-5), ST 34 (Liangqiu), GB 34 (Yanglingquan), SP 9 (Yinlingquan), GB 33 (Xiyangguan), UB 40 (Weizhong), HeDing (EX-LE-2), SP 10 (Xuehai)
- Ankle area: KI 3 (Taixi), UB 62 (Shengmai), KI 6 (Zhaohai), UB 60 (Qunlun), GB 40 (Qiuxu), ST 41 (Jiexi)
- Toe joints: BaFeng (EX-LE-10)
- Xing (Move) Bi syndrome: GB 20 (Fengchi), DU 16 (Fengfu), UB 17 (Geshu), SP 10 (Xuehai), SP 6 (Sanyinjiao)
- Tong (Pain) Bi syndrome: UB 23 (Shenshu), GV 4 (Mingmen), CV 4 (Guanyuan)
- Zhu (Fix) Bi syndrome: ST 36 (Zhusanli), SP 9 (Yinlingquan), SP 5 (Shangqiu)
- Re (Heat) Bi syndrome: GV 14 (Daizhui), LI 11 (Quchi)

Caution

One should wear proper shoes to support the feet and alleviate pressure, reducing the loading from knees and achieving better safety. Avoid risk of joint deformity by using the big joints for tasks, rather than the smaller joints. For example, carrying heavy objects in a back pack is preferable to carrying them by hand in preventing deformity of the fingers. Also, use the palm to exert force when chopping, and use both hands to hold a cup when drinking to avoid heavy loading on the finger joints.

Chapter 38
Coccygeal Pain

Jaung-Geng Lin, Kuen-Bao Chen and Yu-Chen Lee

Coccygeal Pain

1. An unstable coccyx, which causes chronic inflammation
2. A fall or direct trauma to the base of the spine
3. Repetitive strain or overuse, particularly from cycling or rowing
4. Muscle spasm or tightness in the pelvic floor muscles, gluteus maximus, prirformis, or adductor magnus muscles. This pain tends to ease, rather than increase, when sitting
5. Problems following surgery
6. Childbirth

Acupoints

BL 31 (Shangliao), BL 32 (Ciliao), BL 33 (Zhongliao), and BL 34 (Xialia)

Chapter 39
Elbow Pain

Jaung-Geng Lin, Kuen-Bao Chen and Yu-Chen Lee

Symptom 1

Serious pain in the elbow, the arm cannot be rotated, and difficulty lifting things. The tongue body is dark with stasis points, the tongue fur is white and slimy, and the pulse is fine.

Prescription

Following acupuncture points in the elbow are prescribed: LI 12 (Zhuoliao), LI 11 (Quchi), TE 10 (Tianjing), LI 10 (Shousanli), TE 5 (Waiguan), and Ah-Shi.

Operation Method

Use draining method. Intermittently retaining needle for 30 min, and add moxa stick for moxa burning at the same time or use warm acupuncture and moxibustion.

Symptom 2

Elbow pain, which is especially serious at night. The patient is unable to lift heavy things, experiences dizziness, backache, and tinnitus. The tongue is red with less fur, and the pulse is fine and weak.

Prescription

1. BL 18 (Ganshu), BL 23 (Shenshu), BL 17 (Geshu), ST 36 (Zusanli), and SP 6 (Sanyinjiao)
2. LI 12 (Zhuoliao), LI 11 (Quchi), LI 10 (Shousanli), SJ 10 (Tianjing), and Ah-Shi acupuncture points in the elbow

Treatment Method

For the first group of Prescription, tonifying method is used in Shu acupuncture points, retaining needle for 15 min, and moxa stick moxa burning is added.

For the second group of Prescription, neutral supplementation and draining method is used in Shu acupuncture points, moxa stick/moxa burning or warm acupuncture and moxibustion is added, and needle is retained intermittently for 20–30 min.

Chapter 40
Wrist Pain

Jaung-Geng Lin, Kuen-Bao Chen and Yu-Chen Lee

Acupoints

TE 4 (Yangchi), LI 5 (Yangxi), SI 5 (Yanggu)

Methods

Draining method is used. If it is an old injury, retain the needle with moxa stick moxibustion, and the needle is retained for 30 min with hand manipulation at certain intervals. Treat once every day for acute patients and once every other day for chronic patients.

Chapter 41
Ankle Pain

Jaung-Geng Lin, Kuen-Bao Chen and Yu-Chen Lee

Ankle Pain

Ligaments may be injured when a greater than normal stretching force is applied to them. Inversion injuries, in which the foot rolls inward, are more common than eversion injuries (also referred to as a high ankle sprain), where the foot twists outward. Common causes of ankle sprain include:

- Awkward planting the foot when running, stepping up or down, or even performing simple tasks such as getting out of bed.
- Stepping onto an irregular surface, such as stepping into a hole.
- Athletic events where one player may step on another (a common example is a basketball player who goes up for a rebound and comes down on top of another player's foot, causing the rebounder's foot to roll inward).

Acupoints

GB 34 (Yanglingquan), ST 36 (Zusanli), SP 9 (Yinlingquan), GB 40 (Qiuxu), TE 5 (Waiquan)

Chapter 42
Heel Pain

Jaung-Geng Lin, Kuen-Bao Chen and Yu-Chen Lee

Heel pain is most often caused by a condition called plantar fasciitis, sometimes also called heel spur syndrome when a spur is present. Heel pain may also be due to other causes, such as a stress fracture, tendonitis, arthritis, nerve irritation, or, rarely, a cyst.

Because there are several potential causes of heel pain, it is important to have it properly diagnosed. A foot and ankle surgeon can distinguish the difference between the possibilities and determine the underlying cause of the pain.

What Is Plantar Fasciitis?

Plantar fasciitis is an inflammation of the band of tissue (the plantar fascia) that extends from the heel to the toes. In this condition, the fascia first becomes irritated and then inflamed, resulting in heel pain.

K.-B. Chen (✉)
Department of Anesthesiology, China Medical University Hospital,
2 Yuh-Der Road, North District, Taichung, Taiwan 40447, Republic of China
e-mail: d3510@mail.cmuh.org.tw
e-mail: kpc329@yahoo.com.tw

J.-G. Lin
School of Chinese Medicine, China Medical University,
Taichung, Taiwan, Republic of China

Y.-C. Lee
Department of Acupuncture, China Medical University Hospital,
Taichung, Taiwan, Republic of China

Causes

The most common cause of plantar fasciitis is the structure of the foot itself. For example, people who have problems with their arches, either presenting with overly flat or highly-arched feet, will be more prone to developing the condition.

Wearing nonsupportive footwear on hard, flat surfaces puts abnormal strain on the plantar fascia and can also lead to plantar fasciitis. This is particularly evident when one's job requires them to spend long hours on their feet. Obesity may also contribute to plantar fasciitis.

Acupoints

BL 57 (Chengshan), KI 3 (Taixi), BL 60 (Kunlun), BL 58 (Feiyang)

Chapter 43
Insomnia

Jaung-Geng Lin, Kuen-Bao Chen and Yu-Chen Lee

Types of Insomnia

Insomnia may be classified as transient, acute, or chronic.

1. *Transient insomnia* lasts for less than a week. It may be caused by another disorder, by changes in the sleep environment, by the timing of sleep, by severe depression, or by stress. Its consequences—sleepiness and impaired psychomotor performance—are similar to those of sleep deprivation.
2. *Acute insomnia* is the inability to consistently sleep well for a period of less than a month.
3. *Chronic insomnia* lasts for longer than a month. It can be caused by another disorder, or it can be a primary disorder. Its effects can vary according to its causes. They may include muscular fatigue, hallucinations, and/or mental fatigue, but people with chronic insomnia often show increased alertness. Some people living with the disorder report seeing things as if they are happening in slow motion, while moving objects seem to blend together. Chronic insomnia can also cause double vision.

K.-B. Chen (✉)
Department of Anesthesiology, China Medical University Hospital,
2 Yuh-Der Road, North District, Taichung, Taiwan 40447, Republic of China
e-mail: d3510@mail.cmuh.org.tw
e-mail: kpc329@yahoo.com.tw

J.-G. Lin
School of Chinese Medicine, China Medical University,
Taichung, Taiwan, Republic of China

Y.-C. Lee
Department of Acupuncture, China Medical University Hospital,
Taichung, Taiwan, Republic of China

Patterns of Insomnia

Sleep-onset insomnia is the difficulty in falling asleep at the beginning of the night, which is often a symptom of anxiety disorders or the delayed sleep phase disorder. Nocturnal awakenings are characterized by a difficulty in returning to sleep after awakening in the middle of the night or upon waking too early in the morning. Middle-of-the-night insomnia may be a symptom of pain disorders or medical illness, and terminal insomnia is often a characteristic of clinical depression.

Poor Sleep Quality

Poor sleep quality can also occur as a result of other conditions, such as restless legs, sleep apnea, or major depression. Poor sleep quality is caused by the individual not reaching stage 3 or delta sleep, which has restorative properties. There are, however, people who are unable to achieve stage 3 sleep because of brain damage who lead perfectly normal lives.

Major depression leads to alterations in the function of the hypothalamic–pituitary–adrenal axis, causing excessive release of cortisol, which can lead to poor sleep quality. Nocturnal polyuria, excessive nighttime urination, can also be very disturbing to sleep.

Subjective Insomnia

Some cases of insomnia are not really insomnia in the traditional sense. People experiencing sleep state misperception will often sleep for normal durations, yet severely overestimate the time it has taken them to fall asleep. They may believe they have slept for only 4 h, while paradoxically, they have actually slept a full 8 h.

Acupoints

KI 6 (Zhaohai), BL 62 (Shenmai), HT 7 (Shenmen), Ex-HN3 (Yintang), Ex-HN1 (Si Shen Chong)

Chapter 44
Nausea and Vomiting

Jaung-Geng Lin, Kuen-Bao Chen and Yu-Chen Lee

Nausea and vomiting are not diseases, but rather are symptoms of many different conditions, such as infection ("stomach flu"), food poisoning, motion sickness, overeating, blocked intestine, illness, concussion or brain injury, appendicitis, and migraines. Nausea and vomiting can sometimes be symptoms of more serious diseases such as heart attacks, kidney or liver disorders, central nervous system disorders, brain tumors, and some forms of cancer.

What Is the Difference Between Nausea and Vomiting?

Nausea is an uneasiness of the stomach that often accompanies the urge to vomit but does not always lead to vomiting. Vomiting is the forcible voluntary or involuntary emptying ("throwing up") of stomach contents through the mouth. Some triggers that may result in vomiting can come from the stomach and intestines (infection, injury, and food irritation), the inner ear (dizziness and motion sickness), and the brain (head injury, brain infections, tumors, and migraine headaches).

K.-B. Chen (✉)
Department of Anesthesiology, China Medical University Hospital,
2 Yuh-Der Road, North District, Taichung, Taiwan 40447, Republic of China
e-mail: d3510@mail.cmuh.org.tw
e-mail: kpc329@yahoo.com.tw

J.-G. Lin
School of Chinese Medicine, China Medical University,
Taichung, Taiwan, Republic of China

Y.-C. Lee
Department of Acupuncture, China Medical University Hospital,
Taichung, Taiwan, Republic of China

What Causes Nausea or Vomiting?

The causes of nausea and vomiting are quite similar. Many things can bring on nausea. Some common causes are seasickness and other motion sicknesses, early pregnancy, intense pain, exposure to chemical toxins, emotional stress (fear), gallbladder disease, food poisoning, indigestion, various viruses, and certain smells or odors.

The causes of vomiting differ according to age. For adults, vomiting is commonly a result of a viral infection and food poisoning, and occasionally a result of motion sickness and illnesses in which the person has a high fever. For children, it is common for vomiting to occur because of a viral infection, food poisoning, motion sickness, overeating or feeding, coughing, and illnesses in which the child has a high fever. Although rare, blocked intestines can cause vomiting, most typically in early infancy.

Usually vomiting is harmless, but it can be a sign of a more serious illness. Some examples of serious conditions that may bring on nausea or vomiting include concussions, encephalitis, meningitis, intestinal blockage, appendicitis, migraine headaches, and brain tumors.

Another concern with vomiting is dehydration. Adults have a lower risk of becoming dehydrated because they can usually detect the symptoms of dehydration (such as increased thirst and dry lips or mouth). Children have a greater risk of becoming dehydrated, especially if the vomiting occurs with diarrhea, because young children may often be unable to tell an adult about symptoms of dehydration. Adults caring for sick children need to be aware of these visible signs of dehydration: dry lips and mouth, sunken eyes, rapid breathing or pulse, or, in infants, decreased urination and a sunken fontanelle (soft spot on top of the baby's head).

Acupoints

BL 21 (Weishu), CV 13 (Shangwan), CV 12 (Zhongwan), PC 6 (Neiquan), ST 36 (Zusanli)

Chapter 45
Sedation

Jaung-Geng Lin, Kuen-Bao Chen and Yu-Chen Lee

Acupuncture uses in sedation are divided to three parts:

1. Pretreatment for gastroscopy: ST 25 (Tianshu), ST 36 (Zusanli), and ST 37 (Shangjuxu)
2. Electroacupuncture combined with tramadol and midazolam for pain relief during outpatient extracorporeal shockwave lithotripsy: BL 23 (Shenshu), BL 25 (Dachangshu), BL 60 (Kunlun), KI 3 (Taixi), and GB 34 (Yanglingquan)
3. Auricular acupuncture for dental anxiety: relaxation tranquilizer master cerebral point

Chapter 46
Dizziness

Jaung-Geng Lin, Kuen-Bao Chen and Yu-Chen Lee

Dizziness refers to impairment in spatial perception and stability. It is considered imprecise. It can be used to mean vertigo, presyncope, disequilibrium, or for nonspecific feelings such as giddiness or foolishness. One can induce dizziness by engaging in disorientating activities such as spinning.

- Vertigo is a specific medical term used to describe the sensation of spinning or having one's surroundings spin about them. Many people find vertigo very disturbing and often report associated nausea and vomiting. It represents about 25 of cases of occurrences of dizziness.
- Disequilibrium is the sensation of being off balance, and is most often characterized by frequent falls in a specific direction. This condition is not often associated with nausea or vomiting.
- Presyncope is lightheadedness, muscular weakness, and feeling faint as opposed to a syncope, which is actually fainting.
- Nonspecific dizziness is often psychiatric in origin. It is a diagnosis of exclusion and can sometimes be brought about by hyperventilation.

K.-B. Chen (✉)
Department of Anesthesiology, China Medical University Hospital,
2 Yuh-Der Road, North district, Taichung, Taiwan 40447, Republic of China
e-mail: d3510@mail.cmuh.org.tw
e-mail: kpc329@yahoo.com.tw

J.-G. Lin
School of Chinese Medicine, China Medical University,
Taichung, Taiwan, Republic of China

Y.-C. Lee
Department of Acupuncture, China Medical University Hospital,
Taichung, Taiwan, Republic of China

Mechanism

Many conditions cause dizziness because multiple parts of the body are required for maintaining balance, including the inner ear, eyes, muscles, skeleton, and the nervous system.

Common physiological causes of dizziness include the following:

- inadequate blood supply to the brain due to
    a. a sudden fall in blood pressure
    b. heart problems or artery blockages
- loss or distortion of vision or visual cues
- disorders of the inner ear
- distortion of brain/nervous function by medications such as anticonvulsants and sedatives

Acupoints

LI 4 (Hegu), ST 36 (Zusanli), GV 20 (Baihui), SP 9 (Yinlingquan), PC 6 (Neiquan)

Index

5-Hydroxytryptamine (5-HT), 77

A
Abdominal pain, 237
   caution, 238
   treatment, 237
Acupoints, 3
   lineage of, 5, 6
   location of, 6
   stimulation of, 7
Acupuncture, 73, 74, 88, 95, 240
   and moxibustion, 240
   anti-nociceptive effects of, 77, 78
   application of, 101, 103
   benefit of, 89
   chinese theory, 4
   clinical applications of, 81
   clinical efficacy of, 101
   clinical trials of, 90
   definition of, 3
   different forms of, 81
   documentation of, 4
   earliest record of, 87
   early practice, 87
   effectiveness of, 75
   effects of, 74, 81
   efficacy of, 89
   forms of, 102
   Hegu, 229
   hieroglyphs of, 5
   history of, 4, 6
   in sedation, 263
   manual, 81
   manual stimulation, 79
   mechanisms of, 75
   microsystem, 92
   multiple variations of, 87
   origin of, 4
   pain relief, traditional concept of, 7
   postoperative, 113
   practice and teaching of, 88
   relative specificity, 9
   research, 8
   review of, 8
   somatotopic microsystem, 90
   superior analgesic mechanism of, 78
   therapeutic effect of, 8
   therapeutic methods of, 6
   toothache, treatment points, 229
   treatment, 4, 7
Acupuncture analgesia (AA), 81, 102
   anesthesia, 102
   clinical practice of, 8
   decreased, 76
   effects of, 77
   endogenous oipoids, role of, 7
   evidence of, 8
   fMRI study, 8, 9
   history of, 8
   increased, 78
   mechanism of, 7, 73, 74, 78, 80
   recent study, 7
   tolerance of, 7
Acupuncture anesthesia
   development of, 140
Acupuncture assisted anesthesia, 101, 113
Acupuncture needles
   evolution of, 5
Acupuncture points, 74, 87, 153, 241
   14 Daizhui, 177
   Asi Points, 217
   B 16 Muchuang, 196
   Ba Fen, 211
   Ba Xie, 211
   BL 1 Jingming, 179
   BL 2 Cuanzhu, 179

BL 3 Meichong, 179
BL 4 Qucha, 179
BL 5 Wuchu, 179
BL 6 Chengguang, 179
BL 7 Tongtian, 179
BL 8 Luoque, 179
BL9 Yuzhen, 180
BL 10 Tianzhu, 180
BL 11 Dazhu, 180
BL 12 Fengmen, 180
BL 13 Feishu, 180
BL 14 Jueyinshu, 180
BL 15 Xinshu, 180
BL 16 Dushu, 180
BL 17 Geshu, 180
BL 18 Ganshu, 180
BL 19 Danshu, 180
BL 20 Pishu, 180
BL 21 weishu, 180
BL 22 Sanjiaoshu, 180
BL 23 Shenshu, 180
BL 24 Qihaishu, 180
BL 25 Dachangshu, 180
BL 26 Guanyuanshu, 180
BL 27 Xinochaogshu, 180
BL 28 Pangguangshu, 180
BL 29 Zhonglushu, 180
BL 30 Baihuanshu, 181
BL 31 Shangliao, 181
BL 32 Ciliao, 181
BL 33 Zhongliao, 181
BL 34 Xialiao, 181
BL 35 Huiyang, 181
BL 36 Chengfu, 181
BL 37 Yinmen, 181
BL 38 Fuxi, 181
BL 39 Weiyans, 181
BL 40 Weizhong, 181
BL 41 Fufen, 181
BL 42 Pohu, 181
BL 43 Gaohuans, 181
BL 44 Shentang, 181
BL 45 Yixi, 181
BL 46 Geguan, 181
BL 47 Hunmen, 181
BL 48 Yanggang, 181
BL 49 Yishe, 181
BL 50 Weicang, 181
BL 51 Huangmen, 181
BL 52 Zhishi, 183
BL 53 Baohuang, 183
BL 54 Zhibian, 183
BL 55 Heyang, 183

BL 56 Chengjin, 183
BL 57 Chengshan, 183
BL 58 Feiyang, 183
BL 59 Fuyang, 183
BL 60 Kunlun, 183
BL 61 Pushen, 183
BL 62 Shenmai, 183
BL 63 Jinmen, 183
BL 64 Jinggu, 183
BL 65 Shugu, 183
BL 66 Zutonggu, 183
BL 67 zhiyin, 183
conception vessel, 203, 205
CV 1 Huiyin, 203
CV 2 Qugu, 203
CV 3 Zhongji, 203
CV 4 Guanyuan, 203
CV 5 Shimen, 203
CV 6 Qihai, 203
CV 7 Yinjiao, 203
CV 8 Shenque, 203
CV 9 Shuifen, 203
CV 10 Xiawan, 203
CV 11 Jianli, 203
CV 12 Zhongwan, 203
CV 13 Shangwan, 203
CV 14 Juque, 203
CV 15 Jiuwei, 203
CV 16 Zhongting, 203
CV 17 Dhozhong, 203
CV 18 Yutang, 203
CV 19 Zigong, 205
CV 20 Huagai, 205
CV 21 Xuanji, 205
CV 22 Tiantu, 205
CV 23 Lianquan, 205
CV 24 Chengjiang, 205
electrical stimulation of, 81
epigastric pain, treatment, 235
EX-HN1 Si Shen Chong, 211
EX-HN3 Yintang, 211
EX-HN4 Yuyao, 211
EX-HN5 Taiyang, 211
EX-HN6 Erjian, 211
Ex-HN7 Qiuhou, 211
Foot Tai Yin Spleen Meridian, 169–171
Foot Yang Ming Stomach Meridian, 165, 166, 168
for facial nerve palsy, 225
for neck pain, 231
frozen shoulder, 244
GB 1 Tongziliao, 195
GB 2 Tinghui, 195

Index   269

GB 3 Shangguan, 195
GB 4 Hanyan, 195
GB 5 Xuanlu, 195
GB 6 Xuanli, 195
GB 7 Qubin, 195
GB 7 Qubin and GB 5 Xuanlu, 195
GB 8 Shuaigu, 195
GB 9 Tianchong, 195
GB 10 Fubai, 195
GB 11 Touqiaoyin, 196
GB 11 Touqiaoyin and GB 9 Tianchong, 195
GB 12 Wangu, 196
GB 13 Benshen, 196
GB 14 Yangbai, 196
GB 15 Toulinqi, 196
GB 15 Toulinqi and GB 20 Fengchi, 196
GB 16 Muchuang, 196
GB 17 Zhengyins, 196
GB 18 Chegling, 196
GB 19 Naokong, 196
GB 20 Fengchi, 196
GB 20 Fengchi and GB 15 Toulinqi, 196
GB 21 Jianjing, 196
GB 22 Yuanye, 196
GB 23 Zhejin, 196
GB 24 Jihyueh, 196
GB 25 Jingmen, 196
GB 26 Daimai, 196
GB 27 Wushu, 196
GB 28 Weidao, 196
GB 29 Juliao, 196
GB 30 Huantiao, 196
GB 31 Fengshi, 198
GB 32 Zhongdu, 198
GB 33 Xiyangguan, 198
GB 34 Yanglingquan, 198
GB 35 Yangjiao, 198
GB 36 Waichiou, 198
GB 37 Guangming, 198
GB 38 Yangfu, 198
GB 39 Xuanzhong, 198
GB 40 Qiuxu, 198
GB 41 Zulinqi, 198
GB 42 Diwuhui, 198
GB 43 Jiaxi, 198
GB 44 Zuqiaoyin, 198
governor vessel, 207–209
GV-1 Changqian, 207
GV-2 Yaoshu, 207
GV-3 Yaoyangguan, 207
GV-4 Mingmen, 207
GV-5 Xuanshu, 207

GV-6 Zizhong, 207
GV-7 Zhongshu, 207
GV-8 Jinsuo, 207
GV-9 Zhiyang, 207
GV-10 Lingtai, 207
GV-11 Shendao, 207
GV-12 Shenzhu, 207
GV 13 Taodao, 177
GV-13 Taodao, 207
GV-14 DaiZhui, 208
GV 14 Daizhui and acromion, 196
GV-15 Yamen, 208
GV-16 Fengfu, 208
GV-17 Naohu, 208
GV-18 Qiangjian, 208
GV-19 Houdins, 208
GV-20 Baihui, 209
GV-21 Q1anding, 209
GV-22 Xinhui, 209
GV-23 Shangxing, 209
GV-24 Shenting, 209
GV-25 Suliao, 209
GV-26 Shuigou, 209
GV-27 DuiDuan, 209
GV 28 Yinjiao, 209
Hand Sho Yin Heart Meridian, 173
Hand Tai Yin Lung Meridian, 159
Hand Yang Ming Large Intestine Meridian, 161, 162
HT 1 Jiquan, 173
HT 2 Qingling, 173
HT 3 Shaohai, 173
HT 4 Lingdao, 173
HT 5 Tongli, 173
HT 6 Yinxi, 173
HT 7 Shenmen, 173
HT 8 Shaofu, 174
HT 9 Shaochong, 174
HuaTao Jai Ji, 211
KI 1 Yongquan, 185
KI 2 Rangu, 185
KI 3 Taixi, 185
KI 3 (Taixi) and LR 3 (Taichong), 230
KI 4 Dazhong, 185
KI 5 Shuiquan, 185
KI 6 Zhaohai, 185
KI 7 Fuliu, 185
KI 8 Jiaoxin, 187
KI 9 Zhubin, 187
KI 11 Henggu, 187
KI 12 Dahe, 187
KI 13 Qixue, 187
KI 14 Siman, 187

KI 15 Zhonszhu, 187
KI 16 Huangshu, 187
KI 17 shangqu, 187
KI 18 Shiguan, 187
KI 19 Yindu, 187
KI 20 Futonggu, 187
KI 22 Bulang, 187
KI 23 Shenfeng, 187
KI 24 Lingxu, 187
KI 25 Shencang, 187
KI 26 Yuzhong, 187
KIU 21 Youmen, 187
LI 1 Shangyang, 161
LI 2 Erjian, 161
LI 3 Sanjian, 161
LI 4 Hegu, 161
LI 5 Yangxi, 161
LI 6 Pianli, 161
LI 7 Wenliu, 161
LI 8 Xialian, 161
LI 9 Shanglian, 161
LI 10 Shousanli, 161
LI 11 Quchi, 162
LI 12 Zzhouliao, 162
LI 13 Shouwuli, 162
LI 14 Binao, 162
LI 15 Jianyu, 163
LI 16 Jugu, 163
LI 17 Tianding, 163
LI 18 Futu, 163
LI 19 Heliao, 163
LI 20 Yingxiang, 163
locations of, 92
LR 1 Dadun, 199
LR 2 Xingjian, 199
LR 3 Taichong, 199
LR 4 Zhongfeng, 199
LR 5 Ligou, 199
LR 6 Zhongdu, 199
LR 7 Xiguan, 199
LR 8 Ququan, 199
LR 9 Yinbao, 199
LR 10 Zuwuli, 201
LR 11 Yinlian, 201
LR 12 Jimai, 201
LR 13 Zhangmen, 201
LR 14 Qimen, 201
LU 1 Zhongfu, 159
LU 2 Yunmen, 159
LU 3 Tianfu, 159
LU 4 Xiabai, 159
LU 5 Chize, 159
LU 6 Kongzui, 159

LU 7 Lieque, 159
LU 8 Jingqu, 160
LU 9 Taiyuan, 160
LU 10 Yuji, 160
LU 11 Shaoshang, 160
manipulation of, 79
PC 1 Tianchi, 189
PC 2 Tianquan, 189
PC 3 Quze, 189
PC 4 Ximen, 189
PC 5 Jianshi, 189
PC 6 Neiguan, 189
PC 7 Daling, 189
PC 8 Laogong, 190
PC 9 Zhongchong, 190
physical stimulation, 92
Qi Yen, 217
SI 1 Chengqi, 165
SI 1 Shaoze, 175
SI 2 Qiangu, 175
SI 3 Houxi, 175
SI 4 Wangu, 175
SI 5 Yanggu, 175
SI 6 Yanglao, 175
SI 8 Xiaohai, 175
SI 9 Jianzhen, 175
SI 10 Naoshu, 175, 177
SI 11 Tianzong, 177
SI 12 Bingfeng, 177
SI 13 Quyuan, 177
SI 16 Tianchuang, 177
SI 17 Tianrong, 177
SI 18 Quanliao, 177
SI 19 Tinggong, 177
Si Feng, 217
SP 1 Yinbai, 169
SP 2 Dadu, 169
SP 3 Taibai, 169
SP 4 Gongsun, 169
SP 5 Shansqiu, 169
SP 6 Sanyinjiao, 169
SP 7 Logu, 169
SP 8 Diji, 169
SP 9 Yinlingquan, 169
SP 10 Xuehai, 169
SP 11 Jimen, 169
SP 12 Chongmen, 169
SP 13 Fushe, 170
SP 14 Fujie, 170
SP 15 Daheng, 170
SP 16 Fuai, 170
SP 17 Shidou, 171
SP 18 Tianxi, 171

Index

SP 19 Xiongxiang, 171
SP 20 Zhourong, 171
SP 21 Dabao, 171
ST 2 Sibai, 165
ST 3 Juliao, 165
ST 4 Dicang, 165
ST 5 Daying, 165
ST 6 Jiache, 165
ST 7 Xiaguan, 165
ST 8 Touwei, 165
ST 8 Touwei and GB 7 Qubin, 195
ST 9 Renyins, 165
ST 10 Shuitu, 165
ST 11 Qishe, 165
ST 12 Quepen, 165
ST 13 Qihu, 166
ST 14 Kufang, 166
ST 15 Wuyi, 166
ST 16 Yingchuang, 166
ST 17 Ruzhong, 166
ST 18 Rugen, 166
ST 19 Burong, 166
ST 20 Chengman, 166
ST 21 Liangmen, 166
ST 22 Guanmen, 166
ST 23 Taiyi, 166
ST 24 Huaroumen, 166
ST 25 Tianshu, 166
ST 26 wailing, 166
ST 27 Daju, 166
ST 28 Shuidao, 166
ST 29 Guilai, 166
ST 30 Qichong, 166
ST 31 Biguan, 166
ST 32 Futu, 166
ST 33 Yinshi, 166
ST 34 Liangqiu, 166
ST 35 Dubi, 168
ST 36 Zusanli, 168
ST 37 Shangjuxu, 168
ST 38 Tiaokou, 168
ST 39 Xiajuxu, 168
ST 40 Fenglong, 168
ST 41 Jiexi, 168
ST 42 Chongyang, 168
ST 43 xiangu, 168
ST 44 Neiting, 168
ST 45 Lidui, 168
TE 1 Guanchong, 191
TE 2 Yemen, 191
TE 3 Zhongzhu, 191
TE 4 Yangchi, 191
TE 5 Waiguan, 191
TE 6 Zhigou, 191
TE 7 Huizong, 191
TE 8 Sanyangluo, 191
TE 9 Sidu, 191
TE 10 Tianjing, 191
TE 11 Qinglengyuan, 192
TE 12 Xiaoluo, 192
TE 13 Naohui, 193
TE 14 Jianliao, 193
TE 15 Tianliao, 193
TE 16 Tianyu, 193
TE 17 Yifeng, 193
TE 18 Chimai, 193
TE 19 Luxi, 193
TE 20 Jiaosun, 193
TE 21 Ermen, 193
TE 22 Erheliao, 193
TE 23 Sizhukong, 193
traditional, 96
upper back pain, treatment, 241
Yao Tong Dian, 211
Acupuncture practices
  systems of, 92
Acute lumbar sprain
  in lower back pain, 245
Ankle pain, 255
Ankle sprain, 255
Ankylosing spondylitis (AS), 241
Arthritis
  caution, 248
  clinical signs of, 247
  diagnosis of, 247
  treatment, 247, 248
Auricular acupuncture, 143
  adverse effects of, 142
  history of, 139, 140
  methods of, 141
  theory of, 139, 140
  therapy, 139
Auricular diagnosis, 140
Auricular points, 140, 142
  anatomy of, 140
  mapping of, 140
  nomenclature of, 140
Auricular therapy, 143
  in treatment of insomnia, 144
  use of, 144

B

Back and chest pain
  BL13 (Feishu), 233
  RN12 (Zhongwan), 233
  ST40 (Fenglong), 233

Blood, 33
  circulation of, 27, 31, 32
  composition of, 13
  constituents of, 32
  consumption of, 32
  deficiency of, 29, 40
  diseases of, 33
  flow of, 40
  harmanious flow of, 37
  pathology, 33
  production of, 32
  stagnation of, 27, 40
  theory of, 31, 34
Body acupuncture treatment, 222
  acupoints for, 222
  forehead pain, 222
  in dysmenorrhea, 240
Body fluids, 34
  circulation of, 25
  form of, 16
  regulating, 20
  theory of, 31, 34

C
Chest pain, 233
  BI17 (Geshu), 233
  BL14 (Jueyingshu), 233
  BL15 (Xinshu), use, 233
  LR3 (Taichong), 233
  LU5 (Chize), use, 233
  PC6 (Neiguan) use, 233
  RN17 (Danzhong), use, 233
Cholecystokinin octapeptide (CCK), 77
Chronic lumbar strain
  in lower back pain, 245
Chronic patients
  wrist pain, 253
Clinical research
  of lower back pain, 246
Cluster headaches, 222
  occurrence, 222
Coccygeal pain, 249
Connective tissue, 75
Constitutional balance, 103, 106
Cupping, 95
Curious meridian, 106
  treatments, 106
Cutaneous needling method
  for dysmenorrhea, 240
Cyclooxygenase-2 (COX-2), 78

D
Deep tissue nerve fibers, 75
Deficiency syndrome
  vertigo, 227, 228
Dehydration, 262
  symptoms of, 262
Diagnosis
  of frozen shoulder, major points, 243
Direct pressure, 93
Disease causation
  in five-phase theory, 21, 23
  magical explanations, 34
Disequilibrium, 265
Dizziness, 265
  mechanism of, 266
  non-specific, 265
  physiological causes of, 266
Double vision, 259
Draining method
  wrist pain, 253
Duodental ulcers, 237
Dysmenorrhea
  caution, 240,
  clinical research, 240
  cutaneous needling method, 240
  etiology and pathology, 239
  moxibustion therapy, 240
  treatment, 240

E
Ear acupuncture, 139, 223
  in dysmenorrhea, 240
Elbow pain
  operation method, 251
  patient, 252
  prescription, 251, 252
  symptom, 251, 252
  treatment method, 252
Electrical stimulation, 96
  frequency of, 96
  intensity of, 96
Electroacupuncture (EA), 74, 76, 78, 81
  duration of, 81
  frequencies of, 76
  high frequency, 78
  lower frequency, 78
Electroacupuncture stimulations (EAS), 96
Endogenous, 35
Epigastric pain, 235
  clinical investigation, 235
Essence, 33
  postnatal, 33
  prenatal, 32

Index

secondary store of, 33
storage of, 20
Etiology and pathology
    frozen shoulder, 243
Eversion injuries, 255
Excessive nighttime urination, 260
Excessive sexual activity, 35, 41
Excess syndrome
    vertigo, 228
Exogenous, 35

F
Facial nerve palsy
    acupuncture points for, 225
    draining method, 225
    treatment, 225
Five phases, 14, 18, 23
    controlling cycles, 21
    engendering cycles, 21
    in therapeutics, 22
Food poisoning, 262
Foot Jun Yin Liver Meridian
    acupuncture points, 199, 201
Foot Shao Yang Gall Bladder Meridian
    acupuncture points, 195, 196, 198
Foot Shao Yin Kidney Meridian
    acupuncture points, 185, 187
Foot Tai Yang Bladder Meridian
    acupuncture points, 179–181, 183
Foot-Taiyang meridian, 231
Frozen shoulder, 243
    caution, 244
    clinical signs of, 243
    patients with, 243
    treatment, 244
Functional dysmenorrheal\t see Primary
        dysmenorrhea, 239
Functional magnetic resonance imaging
        (fMRI), 8
    acupuncture-related, 8
    studies, 79, 80

G
General linear model (GLM), 79

H
Hand and Foot Yangming
    meridians of, 229
Hand Jue Yin Pericardium Meridian
    acupuncture points, 189
Hand Sho Yang Triple Energizer Meridian
    acupuncture points, 191, 193

Hand Tai Yang small intestine meridian
    acupuncture points, 175, 177
Heel pain, 257
    causes of, 258
    potential causes of, 257
    resulting in, 257
    treatment, 258
Heel spur syndrome, 257
Hegu, 229
    toothache pain, treatment, 229
Hemorrhage, 240
History
    acupuncture analgesia, 8
Hydroinjection, 96

I
Improper diet, 40
    lifestyle factors, 40
Increased menstrual flow, 239
Independent component analysis (ICA), 79
Insomnia
    acute, 259
    cases of, 260
    chronic, 259
    patterns of, 260
    subjective, 260
    transient, 259
    treatment of, 260
    types of, 259
Integrated facet syndrome
    in lower back pain, 245
Integrated lumbar transverse process
        syndrome
    in lower back pain, 245
Inter-consuming-supporting
    yinyang theory, 17
Interdependence
    yinyang theory, 16, 17
Intermittent colic, 239
Inter-transforming
    yinyang theory, 17
Inversion injuries, 255

J
Joint pain
    treatment of, 247, 248

L
Laser acupuncture, 97
    efficacy of, 97
Lower back pain
    caution, 246

fewer incidences of, 245
soft tissue, pathological lesion of, 245
superior cluneal nerves, damage, 245
supraspinous and interspinous ligaments, injury, 245
treatment, 246
Lumbar intervertebral disc
in lower back pain, 246
Lumbar pain
patient with, 246

M
Menstrual pain, 239
Mental overexertion, 35
Meridian of Hand and Foot Yangming
facial nerve palsy, treatment for, 225
meridian of Hand-Yangming Hegu
in toothache, 229
Meridians, 4, 87
blockages in, 93
description of, 92
lineage of, 5, 6
number of, 6
original, 6
true nature of, 7
Microsystem
acupuncture, 92
somatotopic, 92
Migraine headaches
factors, 221
patients with, 221
period, 221
precursor symptoms, 221
Miscellaneous, 35
excessive sexual activity, 35
Motion sickness
result of, 262
Moxibustion, 3, 95
burns, 97
evidence of, 5
history of, 6
origins of, 4
therapeutic methods, 6
therapy for dysmenorrhea, 240
Muscle tissue, 75

N
Nausea, 261
causes of, 262
symptoms of, 261
Neck pain
acupuncture points, 231
qi therapy, 231
treatment, 231
Needle, 94, 95
Neiting
toothache pain, treatment, 229
Nervous system, 266
N-methyl-D-aspartic acid (NMDA) receptor, 77
Nocturnal awakenings, 260
Nocturnal polyuria, 260
Nonpenetrating sham acupuncture (NPSA), 81

O
Obesity, 258
Opioids, 76, 77
Opposition
yinyang theory, 15
Overstrain injuries
in lower back pain, 245

P
Pain
in cluster headaches, 222
Pain fibers, 75, 76
Pain relief
acupuncture needles, 5
Partial dislocation
in lower back pain, 245
Pathogenic factors
endogenous, 35
exogenous, 35
miscellaneous, 35, 39
secondary, 35
TCM classification of, 35
Patients, 239
Percutaneous electroacupoint stimulations (PEAS), 96
Physical overexcretion, 35
Piriformis muscle syndrome
in lower back pain, 245
Plantar fasciitis, 257
common cause of, 258
Poor sleep
excessive nighttime urination, 260
nocturnal polyuria, 260
Poor sleep quality, 260
hypothalamic-pituitary-adrenal axis, function, 260
Positron emission tomography (PET)
studies, 80
Postoperative acupuncture, 113
Postoperative nausea and vomiting (PONV)
treatment of, 144
Pre-operative preparation, 103, 107
constitutional balance, 103
curious meridians, 106

Index

Press needle, 141
Pressure pain detection thresholds (PPDT), 81
Presyncope, 265
Primary dysmenorrhea, 239
   symptoms of, 239
Proximal interphalangeal (PIP) joint, 154

Q

Qi, 31
   chest, 32
   circulation of, 25
   concept of, 31
   counter-flow, 33
   defensive, 33, 34
   deficiency of, 32, 40
   descending of, 20
   disturbances of, 37
   flow of, 20, 27, 35, 37, 38, 40, 153
   generalized deficiency, 41
   movement of, 37
   nutritive, 32
   obstruction of, 32
   original, 32
   pathology of, 33
   sinking, 33
   stagnation of, 33, 41
   theory of, 31, 34
   unimpeded flow of, 27
Qi therapy
   neck pain, 231

R

Rheumatic arthritis (RA), 241

S

Scapular spine
   SI 9 Jianzhen in depression inferior, 175
Sciatica
   in lower back pain, 245
Secondary Dysmenorrhea, 239
Second thoracic vertebrae, 177
Sedation
   dental anxiety, auricular acupuncture for, 263
   electroacupuncture, 263
   gastroscopy, pretreatment for, 263
   parts of, 263
Senile kyphosis, 241
Sensory fibers, 74
Sho-Yin couplets, 153
Shu acupuncture points
   tonifying method, 252
Sleep-onset insomnia, 260
Soreness
   in frozen shoulder, 243
Spinning, 265
Sprain injury of joints
   in lower back pain, 245
Stimulation techniques, 93, 96
   cupping, 95
   direct pressure, 93
   electrical stimulation, 96
   hydroinjection, 96
   moxibustion, 95
   needle, 94, 95
Stomach meridian
   ST36, 237
Supra-spinous fossa
   SI 10 Naoshu, 177

T

Tai-Yang couplets, 153
Tension headaches, 222
   onset of, 222
the\Mother-Son\ relationship
   disease causation, 21
   engendering cycle, 19
Theory of channels and collaterals, 30, 34
Theory of the viscera and bowels, 23, 30
Toothache
   Meridian of Hand-Yangming Hegu, 229
   treatment of, 229
Traditional Chinese Medicine (TCM), 34, 39, 41, 88
   aspect of, 18
   basic theories of, 14
   philosophy of, 73
   practice of, 41
   principles of, 93
   theoretical framework of, 14
   vital substances of, 31
Transcutaneous electrical nerve stimulation (TENS), 96
Treatment
   for body acupuncture, 222
   for chest pain, 233
   for ear acupuncture, 223
   for facial nerve palsy, 225
   of abdominal pain, 237

U

Upper back pain
   acupuncture prescription, 241
   causes of, 241
   caution, 242
   treatment, 241, 242

V

Vertigo, 227, 265
  acupuncture point selection with, 228
  clinical manifestation, 227
  deficiency syndrome, 227, 228
  excess syndrome, 228
  symptoms of, 227
  syndrome differentiation and treatment, 227, 228
  treatment, 228
Viral infection, 262
Vital substances, 31
  blood, 33
  body fluids, 34
  body's stores of, 31
  essence, 33
  interaction of, 31
  of TCM, 31
  qi, 31, 33
Vomiting, 261
  causes of, 262
  symptoms of, 261
  treatment of, 262

W

Warm acupuncture and moxibustion, 251
Wrist pain
  acupoint, 253
  chronic patients, 253
  draining method, 253

Y

Yang-Ming couplets, 153
Yinyang, 14
  balance, 37
  concepts of, 15
  interdependence of, 16, 29
  inter-transformation of, 17
Yinyang theory, 14, 18
  inter-consuming-supporting, 17
  interdependence, 16
  inter-transforming, 17
  opposition, 15

Milton Keynes UK
Ingram Content Group UK Ltd.
UKHW052208150424
441181UK00015B/83